SWINGERS

'And, is it what you expected?' Larry presses. 'Is this how you imagined your Anita would look while she's kissing another woman?'

Damien watches Cora and Anita for a moment longer before responding.

Anita's blouse is open. Cora has a hand inside and whatever it is her fingers are doing the movement is exciting both women. Anita continues to touch Cora's thinly veiled breasts while their mouths join in a slippery union of passion. Together they are panting and hungrily pressing into each other.

'I never thought we'd get to do this,' Damien says eventually.

Cora pulls her face from Anita's lips and looks kindly at him. 'You'll both get to do a lot more before the night's over.' She glances slyly at Larry and then adds, 'At least,you will if you're up for it.'

SWINGERS

Ashley Lister

First published in 2006 by
Virgin Books
Thames Wharf Studios
Rainville Rd
London W6 9HA

A catalogue record of this book is available from the British
Library

ISBN 0 7535 1135 5
ISBN 9 780753 511350

Design and typesetting by TW Typesetting, Plymouth, Devon
Printed and bound by Bookmarque Ltd

CONTENTS

Introduction

S winging is a lot like watching soap operas: so many people do it but so few will ever admit that they do.

For the purposes of this book, swinging is a blanket term used to cover those incidents within relationships where established couples consent to their partners having sexual encounters with others. These encounters range from mild flirtations, kissing and exhibitionism through to full penetrative sex, orgies, dogging and gangbangs.

Swinging and the terms threesomes, foursomes and moresomes are all synonyms for the same phenomenon that has crept stealthily across Western culture over the past sixty years. Originally referred to as 'wife-swapping', swinging is the term currently deemed politically correct because it suggests less of a patriarchal establishment and reflects the easy-going attitude of those involved in this alternative lifestyle.

Swingers come in all shapes and sizes, incorporated in a demograph that ranges from the age of consent up to and beyond retirement. Religion, race, political views and financial status do not bar anyone from participating. Proponents of recreational sex come from all walks of life and, in the UK, they reside in each corner of all four countries.

However, the most remarkable aspect about swinging is not its broad popularity across all social boundaries but that acknowledgement of its occurrence remains virtually non-existent. Occasionally, a Sunday newspaper will provide a damning exposé on a small clique of swingers and shock its scandalised readers with lurid details of what occurs in such dens of iniquity. Or a tabloid might decry a heinous villainess and use an incidence of troilism as proof of her subversive nature. But, aside from the occasional salacious documentary, the swinging lifestyle is usually overlooked, ignored or forgotten.

Swingers do not get mentioned in soap operas, our society's barometer of every acceptable and unacceptable social interaction. Soaps will gladly tackle spousal abuse, drug cultures, murder, incest, interracial relationships and transsexualism. But none of them has ever shown a content swinging couple.

According to Isaac Asimov, 'Jokes of the proper kind, properly told, can do more to enlighten questions [. . .] than any number of dull arguments.' Yet there are no jokes specifically about swingers. There are jokes covering every other topic in the universe, and there are a vast number of jokes about sex and sexuality. But none specifically about the swinging community.

Nearly every other sexual proclivity is covered. 'I had a friend who was into necrophilia, flagellation and bestiality. I always thought he was flogging a dead horse.' Or, 'The masochist says to the sadist, "Hurt me! Hurt me!" and the sadist says, "No!"'

There are jokes about virgins, newlyweds, old married couples, adulterous couples, men with large penises, men with small penises, men with no penises. There are jokes about women with huge breasts, large bottoms, wide and gaping vaginas and every other variation on the human anatomy.

But there are no jokes exclusively about swingers.

Usually, especially here in the UK where we are renowned for our sense of humour, when we know about a subject we make jokes. Considering the vacuum of comedy surrounding the subject, swinging must truly be an unknown commodity.

Agony aunts and those sensational talk-show hosts who occasionally brush on the topic of swinging persistently treat the subject with a disparaging undertone. They claim a third person in the bedroom is a sign that things are about to deteriorate and the prospect of pairing off with another couple is symptomatic of deviance in its most unpleasant form. But, while it does happen that some swinging encounters end badly, a good number of them conclude so satisfactorily that they allow another couple to enter the elite group of hedonists known as swingers.

The purpose of this book is to show that swinging is now more popular than ever and to illustrate some of the ways in which it is currently practised. The stories come from active participants in today's swinging scene who have spoken openly about their activities and I have only changed their names to maintain their anonymity. However, anonymous or not, without their candid contributions this book would not have been possible and I would like to thank them all for taking the time to share an intimate part of their lives.

WHAT IS SWINGING?

swinging (adj.) **1**. sexually promiscuous. **2**. practising exchange of partners, especially spouses, for sex.

S winging means different things to different people and will never be defined by something as dry as a dictionary definition. The consensus amongst those interviewed in the process of making this book suggests that swinging is the ultimate act of sexual freedom between loving and open-minded partners.

The arguments in favour of swinging are compelling. Recreational sex between two or more consenting adults should be an erotically charged experience. As Woody Allen quipped, 'Sex between two people is a beautiful thing – between five it's fantastic.' Or, equally appropriate, 'Sex between a man and a woman can be absolutely wonderful, provided you get between the right man and the right woman.'

Because swinging can incorporate a broad spectrum of fetishes, deviations and tastes, it is open to anyone who wants to participate. The swinging lifestyle allows women to explore their bisexuality; encourages men to viscerally enjoy their partner's pleasure; and (according to its exponents) promotes greater levels of honesty within existing relationships.

Scientifically, it has been argued that men and women were genetically designed to enjoy group sex and multiple partners. According to the results of a Baker and Bellis study of cohabiting students at the University of Manchester, only a small percentage of the sperm released in a 'normal' ejaculate are intended for procreation. The majority are the equivalent of a 'sperm militia', carried along in the ejaculate with the express purpose of destroying any other sperm they encounter within the vaginal canal. Their natural function and the fact that these antagonistic sperm are much more copious when a male suspects his partner has been with another lover suggest the human male is designed to indulge in procreation with a naturally promiscuous mate. The ejaculation of these greater numbers is always more forceful and provides the male with a stronger and more satisfying orgasm. The findings of this survey would suggest that sex for the male of a swinging couple is a far more intense experience than for one who doesn't swing and has a monogamous partner. Similar surveys indicate the female propensity for multiple orgasms is best exploited by group sex. Researchers have also found that females having unprotected sex with more than one partner are able to subconsciously choose the moment of orgasm, allowing them a degree of choice in which partner's sperm is favoured with entry into the cervix. If the results of these investigations are to be accepted and believed, it does imply humans have evolved to enjoy swinging.

Religious arguments are never simplistic and, while the Bible does say *love thy neighbour*, few would seriously argue this statement advocates wife-swapping on any level. Yet many swingers maintain strong religious beliefs and balance this faith with their accepting attitudes towards recreational sex. They sincerely love their spouses; they enjoy the pleasure of sharing, having multiple partners and indulging in group sex; and they devoutly adhere to their interpretation of their religious beliefs. The majority marry these conflicting ideals with the simple knowledge that they are not committing a sin: they have simply taken their relationship to an unconventional level of pleasure and honesty.

Sociologists suggest swingers are drawn by the community aspect of recreational sex, citing friendships that developed as a bonus to the sex, or sex that developed as a bonus to the friendship.

Anthropologists draw comparisons between swingers and the bonobo, a species of primates with a society that revolves around group sex. They explain (the anthropologists, not the primates) that the bonobos set a precedent in their relationships that shows human swingers are not doing anything that isn't natural in at least one part of the animal world.

But, rather than restate the opinions of 'experts' who are only trying to prove their personal hypotheses, this book has been written after interviewing those actively involved in swinging today. It is the author's belief that genuine swingers can better explain the attraction of the phenomena and more easily describe its benefits, drawbacks and (of course) its pleasures.

Andrew, Brenda & Charlie
'Sex is only ever about sex.'

B renda steps into the room with Andrew holding her right arm and Charlie on her left. At any other function, the two men would be assumed to be close acquaintances: a partner and a friend, siblings, cousins or work colleagues. But here everyone understands Brenda is accompanied by her two lovers.

She admits that it is a liberating position. Having a man on each arm makes her feel as though she is adored.

The room has been made small by the dozen or so couples already there. Everyone is dressed in the latest styles and fashions and it is clear that each individual has invested many hours of preparation before attending. The gentlemen wear razor-sharp creases, polished shoes and designer shirts so new they still smell like their original packaging. The ladies bask in a post-hairstylist glow and look as though they have won a date with their favourite movie idol.

Music from the 80s pounds through gargantuan speakers at either end of the room. Tracks from Michael Jackson's *Thriller*, the Human League's *Dare*, and Soft Cell's *Non Stop Erotic Cabaret* follow each other from the CD's random interchanger. The bass rhythms tremble through the laminated floor and make conversation impractical if not impossible.

Two couples sit on either side of a sumptuous settee. They are close together, kissing and holding each other intimately. A small crowd is gathered around the table in the corner from where the drinks are being served. One pair, seemingly oblivious to everyone else, dance together in the centre of the room. Others, scattered around the various corners, lean close together to make their whispers heard over the roar of 'Love Action'.

Andrew kisses Brenda lightly before extracting his arm and going to get refreshments for the three of them. Brenda sees a couple she knows from previous parties and saunters over to greet them. Charlie remains gallantly at her side and is included in the polite introductions.

Andrew: 'Unless you've been to a party, it's impossible for you to know what it's like. Everyone thinks a swing party is a sexual free-for-all, and that you just turn up at the door with an erection and get instantly laid.' He laughs at the notion, shakes his head and says, 'Nothing could be further from the truth.'

Andrew and Brenda are 32 and 29, respectively. They have been married for five years and swinging for two.

'The protocol for swinging parties is more rigid than you'd find at a Victorian tea party,' Andrew explains. 'You can't get in if you're a single man. Men and women are expected to remain in very close proximity to their partners throughout the evening. It's not done to get drunk. But there's always alcohol available. Drugs are a big no-no, although we've been to a couple of parties where I've seen couples passing round a dodgy roll-up or two. And you don't touch anyone unless they invite you to touch them. Also, in a lot of cases, you're expected to be psychic. If a couple are getting it on, you should only watch if they want you to watch. After you've chatted with another couple, and introduced yourself, you're meant to understand what they're into from a conversation that's lost under all the music, with a meaning that's hidden behind euphemism, embarrassment and uncertainty.' Elaborating, he says, 'Brenda and I know what we want and we understand each other's limits. But a lot of couples come to these parties after having some vague conversation that confirms they want to "do it" with another couple. They might be one of those intuitive couples who understand exactly what each other means when they say they want to "do it" with another couple. More often than not, they've both turned up with different expectations. He wants to watch her lezz off with some lass who looks like Pamela Anderson; she fancies the idea of either the softest of soft swaps or, at the other end of the spectrum, she wants a full-blown DP with a pussy to munch on as she comes.' Laughing again, he adds, 'With so much weighted against the chances, it's a wonder anyone ever gets laid at a swing party. But it does happen. Nearly always: it happens.'

With Charlie properly introduced to the other couple, and Andrew returned and having distributed drinks, Brenda leads the conversation. She is a tall lady, her pale skin made lighter by the black dress she wears this evening. Her brunette hair is tied back from her angular face to show perfectly applied lipstick and eyeliner. She is confident and tactile in her gestures and, now she is in the sanctuary of the party, Brenda is bereft of reservations. 'I hear that pubes are coming back into vogue this season,' she tells the other woman. 'The prepubescent look is becoming tired.'

'Couldn't you have phoned me to let me know that?' The other woman giggles. Her husband, beside her, smiles perfunctorily. 'I spent two hours in the bathroom tweezing out every last hair this afternoon,' she complains. 'It was like self-inflicted sadomasochism.'

'You'll have to show me the results,' Brenda says and smiles.

'You can feel them,' the other woman replies encouragingly. She reaches for Brenda's empty left hand and guides it between her thighs. Because the other woman is wearing a short skirt, and not wearing panties, Brenda's fingers slip against smooth, freshly shaved flesh.

The party continues around them. 'Love Action' is replaced by Soft Cell's 'Frustration'. The dancing couple in the centre of the room have been joined by another pair. The more observant members of the party might have noticed that the first couple are no longer dancing with their original partners, although it is unlikely anyone will care. A pall of equanimity cloaks the room's mood and the prevalent attitude is clearly one of laissez-faire. All four writhe their hips and sashay around the impromptu dance floor while challenging each other via mesmerising gazes.

Another couple enter the room, apologising for being late. Someone latches on to the comment and makes a joke about the perils of coming too quickly. A flutter of high-pitched laughter draws attention to the nervousness underpinning events. The chatter of conversation reaches a volume that fights against the pounding of Soft Cell. On the settee, the couples furthest from the door exchange a long, lingering kiss.

Brenda slides her fingers easily over the woman's bald pussy lips. Their gazes remain interlocked and each struggles to appear calm and unmoved by the exchange. At any other party it would be unthinkable for two women to enjoy such a bold interplay in full view of all the other guests. Here, even though it is supposed to be the norm, it is early enough in the evening for the act to be viewed as daring.

However, Brenda does like to be seen as daring.

'That feels lovely,' Brenda sighs. She doesn't take her hand away. Instead, her fingers continue to tease the woman's sex lips. The flesh is warm and moist. 'How did you really get yourself so smooth?'

'I was being serious with what I said before. I used tweezers.'

They both wince. The conversation moves on to depilation products. Brenda sympathises with the woman's problem. She has luxuriant, thick, dark hair; shaving leaves an uncomfortable stubble; she has yet to find a hair removal cream that is safe for the skin around her pubic region while still effective against the hairs.

And Brenda still doesn't take her hand away. She has already ingratiated a finger between the woman's pussy lips and slipped it inside. The moist hole clutches tight around the tip of her middle finger.

The men around them exchange polite glances and nods of unspoken greeting. The lack of conversation between them is universally understood as acceptable while they all watch the two women become acquainted.

Brenda passes her drink to Charlie, leaving her right hand free. Her new friend follows her example and passes her Becks to her husband. No longer encumbered by bottles or glasses, they assume a more natural position together so they can kiss and touch and explore.

Andrew: 'People outside swinging just don't understand what really happens at a party. Don't you get jealous? Do you get much pussy? Is your wife some sort of slut? The questions say as much about their own problems as they could ever reveal about any aspect of swinging. Yes, I sometimes get jealous. But not in a bad way. Brenda and I don't go to parties to hurt each other. We go to have fun. Do I get much pussy? It depends how you define "much". At some parties I might have sex with two, three or four women. At others I might not have sex with anyone. It all depends how the evening pans out. It's not like you buy a ticket on the door that entitles you to four fucks in an evening, and you go from one woman to another until you've had your ticket stamped the appropriate number of times.

'Is my wife some sort of slut? My wife and I share a relationship where we can be open and honest about our sexual needs. She has a demanding libido and I wouldn't be able to fully satisfy her without the swinging aspect of our lives. That means, without the swinging, either Brenda would be frustrated or possibly cheating on me. With the swinging, it means that Brenda is satisfied and we have the advantage of being wholly honest with each other. Some people might describe her as being a slut because of that. But people always give stupid names to things when they don't understand them. I believe, a lot of the time, when guys make comments like that it's because they really wish they were doing something like this with their wives.'

Brenda and her new friend are pressed into a corner of the room. Their mouths have joined together, Brenda's left breast is being squeezed and she has yet to move her fingers from the shaved lips of the other woman's pussy. Their kiss has the urgent fullness of genuine passion. Neither is going for the faux feminine exchanges shown in so many pornographic movies. Rather than keeping their faces apart and rubbing the tips of their extended tongues together, Brenda and her friend are squashing their lips against each other and enjoying the full thrill of exploration.

Around them the party slowly gathers momentum. Soft Cell's 'Frustration' is replaced by Michael Jackson's 'Beat It'. The heavy bass of the stereo now causes the laminate floor to throb. Six figures gyrate in the centre of the room. One woman is already topless and beginning to ease out of her skirt. Her striptease is encouraged by a slow, approving handclap. She slips her thumbs into the waistband of her skirt and begins to slide the garment down to reveal the whisper of fabric that is her thong.

Sharp words are exchanged in the room's doorway. Someone makes an exclamation, ending with the words, 'I don't fucking think so!' Before anyone can see who is angry, or why, the door has slammed closed and there is one less couple at the party. The momentary silence that ensues is quickly banished by resumed conversations and a handful of sympathetic smiles. Veteran partygoers understand that swinging is not for everyone and sometimes the adventure doesn't always work out as hoped.

Someone lights a cigarette and is immediately told to take it outside. The party's hostess is not allowing smoking on this occasion. The smoker apologises and leaves the room with her partner. A second couple follow them and those who have been to previous parties suspect the two couples will probably have their own smokers' party outside in the garden.

Brenda: 'It's not about sex. It's about eroticism. I don't go to parties so I can get laid by X number of men or X number of women, although, I admit, that's a bonus. But I go to swing parties so I can feel erotic. I go to parties so that I can confirm I'm desirable, and so I can meet other people who are also desirable. I'm not saying that I have issues about how people perceive me, or that Andrew and Charlie aren't enough to satisfy me. I'm just saying that I go because I like meeting people who share my ideas of what constitutes a good time.'

The decision to try swinging was a natural extension of Brenda and Andrew's love life. They met, became lovers, moved in together and then married. They enjoyed a full sex life, constantly experimenting with new ideas and repeatedly rediscovering what the other liked.

'But we were in danger of running out of new ideas,' Brenda explains. 'We'd tried every act that two consenting adults could possibly try and, although it was still fun, I think we both knew it was soon going to turn into a humdrum routine. There isn't a position we haven't tried or a style of sex that we haven't attempted. We've tried bondage, S&M, role-playing and every other variation you can think of. We've done anal, oral, watersports and experimented with various fetishes. We used a lot of fantasy talk in our lovemaking, and a repeated theme was the idea of being with other people. It seemed only natural to change that fantasy into a reality.'

The party has now developed into something bacchanalian. The couple on the settee, who have been kissing, are now on the brink of intercourse. She has released his erection from his pants. He has exposed her breasts and raised her skirt to reveal she is not wearing panties. They glide closer to each other as they continue to kiss and murmur words of approval and encouragement. It is unclear whether they are oblivious to the party that is happening around them, or spurred on by the knowledge that others are close by and might be watching. The only thing that is certain is that both are involved in the excitement of the moment.

The woman who performed the striptease to Michael Jackson's 'Beat It' is now on her knees and sucking between her partner's legs. The gossamer thong she wears displays her backside. The sliver of white cotton trails between the cheeks of her buttocks, over a tautly puckered anus and down to a crotch that has been dampened by her excitement. As she sucks and slurps, her hips continue to sway to the music. Occasionally, she moves her head and puts her mouth over the sheathed erection of the man sitting next to her partner. Her lips are wet with saliva and twisted into a smile of mischievous devilment.

Another couple have left the room to join the smokers who do appear to be having their own party in the house's back garden. Giggles and throaty sighs from outside can be heard in the silences each time the CD's track changes. Eventually, the hostess goes to investigate and make sure the smokers are not running a risk of upsetting her neighbours.

An occasional glass clinks from the nearly forgotten drinks table. The majority of those at the party are now too involved with their various exchanges to be bothered about refreshments.

Brenda: 'Of course, wanting to swing and getting into swinging are two completely different things. We did the whole "talk it through" scenario. We discussed jealousy, disease and danger, and all those other subjects that make swinging sound so fucking awful. The strange thing was, the more we discussed things, the more it seemed like swinging was right for us.

'Stripped naked, Andrew's biggest fear was that we would stop loving each other. I assured him that wasn't going to happen because I love him for who he is: not what happens in the bedroom. My biggest fear was that Andrew wouldn't be able to handle watching me with other men.' She smiles at the memory and explains, 'I obviously didn't know him very well if I thought that would repulse him. It's turned out to be one of his biggest turn-ons.'

Brenda and her new friend continue to kiss. With the exception of their matching black stockings, their clothes and exotic lingerie have been discarded. They cling together in a compression of breasts against breasts and legs wrapped around thighs. Beads of perspiration make them look as though they've just stepped from a shower. In the muted lights of the party's main room, their bare bodies glisten in bronzed splendour. Fingers from both women explore and invade the other. Their gasps are urgent, breathless and passionate. Pushing herself away, finally breaking the intimacy of their lingering kiss, Brenda moves her lips to the other woman's breast and begins to suckle.

Things progress quickly. The other woman's partner touches his wife on the shoulder. She looks, at first, startled by his caress. When she remembers he is in close attendance, she quickly solicits Brenda's approval, and then encourages him to join them. Caught up in the moment, Brenda summons Andrew and Charlie to her assistance. Within seconds, the five are in various states of undress and joined in a mêlée of near-naked passion.

The other woman is taken from behind by her husband. Brenda continues to kiss her new friend, constantly stroking the woman's body and paying homage to her bare flesh. Andrew suckles against his wife's breasts, combining his tongue, lips and teeth in the way he knows she likes best. Charlie stands behind Brenda and plunges into her sex from behind. Occasional compliments are passed back and forth. Brenda tells the woman she is beautiful. Andrew and Charlie bestow the same praise on Brenda. The other couple exchange their own intimate accolades. But the majority of sounds are little more than pleasurable sighs and urgent, demanding grunts. Most of the cries are lost beneath Michael Jackson singing 'Human Nature'.

One couple watch them. They have already sated their passion on the settee and lie in each other's embrace touching in anticipation of another bout of lovemaking.

The climactic cries from outside suggest the smokers and their friends are enjoying their own annexed version of the party. In the centre of the room, the dancing has stopped and two couples lie side by side on the uncomfortable laminate floor. At first glance, it is impossible to say which person arrived with which partner. At second glance, it is obvious that no one is troubled by such a consideration.

Brenda: 'Our first swinging experience came from a contact ad. We'd made up our mind that we were going to do it, so I put an ad in the classified section of *Forum* and sat back and waited for the replies.' She laughs again and shakes her head. 'That's not entirely true. I couldn't just sit back. The idea excited me and frightened me. Every time I thought about it, I nearly cacked my knickers and then I had to go and have a wank. If Andrew was around I'd pounce on him and have a vigorous comfort fuck.

'I got worse when the replies started to come through. And, when we organised our first meet, I was cacking bricks. I wanted to do it – I was so horny to experience Andrew and another guy I was *really* wanting to do it – but because it was such a big step into the unknown I was very, very scared.'

The couple say little about their first experience. The gentleman was clean and presentable, and he helped to provide a sexually satisfying climax to the evening. But, afterwards, he seemed anxious to leave and made no suggestion about future meetings. Andrew was worried that they had committed some social faux pas. Brenda fretted that he hadn't found her sufficiently attractive.

The second time they planned to invite a third party into their bedroom they were less worried about the sex and more concerned about whether their visitor would simply disappear at the end of the night.

'But swinging is like that,' Brenda explains. 'It's different folk looking for different things. Some people are just in it for the sex. Others want a social connection. As well as the sex, I think we were looking for someone who would "click" with us. But it was only when we found Charlie that we realised we'd found what we were looking for.'

Charlie and Andrew throw their used condoms into a plastic-lined waste paper bin that sits discreetly in the corner of the bathroom. They left Brenda to kiss her new friend farewell before allowing the other couple to mingle with the rest of the party. A busty woman in her early thirties, displaying a trim figure adorned with the latest Ann Summers fashions, bursts into the bathroom and presses herself between them to dispose of a used condom. Her hair is a stylised red that looks as though it was coloured earlier in the day. All three of them gather around the bathroom's sink to wash their hands. Charlie recognises the woman from a previous party and reintroduces himself and Andrew. Intimate embraces are exchanged. As she kisses each of the men her breasts crush obviously against their bare chests. To avoid the risk of social embarrassment she reminds them that her name is Lynne.

Lynne was the first of the party to be exiled outside with her cigarettes and she asks Andrew and Charlie if they would care to join her in the back garden.

'Isn't it cold outside?' Charlie asks.

Lynne confides, 'We've found a way to keep each other warm.' With a suggestive smile, she promises she will reveal the secret if they join her.

Charlie politely declines the invitation – Brenda is alone downstairs and he enjoys playing the role of an attentive lover – but Andrew is happy to accept Lynne's offer and the pair go off together.

Downstairs, he discovers Brenda is now in the centre of the settee and enjoying the attention of a round-faced man and his waiflike oriental wife. The sight is sexually exciting. Brenda is only wearing her stockings but her body is modestly covered by the hands and arms of the couple sandwiching her. The oriental woman's fingers play against the split of Brenda's pussy while the man has reached across her body to knead and tease her breasts. Brenda lazily turns her face from one to the other and enjoys being kissed by him, then her and then him again.

After pouring himself a soft drink, Charlie decides to follow Andrew and Lynne to the smokers' party.

Charlie: 'I'm Brenda's lover. I don't know how else to describe myself in the context of our relationship. She's married to Andrew; I live with the pair of them, and I often have sex with her. But try putting all that into the little box you find on forms where it asks for marital status.'

Charlie is younger than Andrew and Brenda by a couple of years. Whereas Andrew has an athletic build, Charlie looks more like a construction worker. His biceps are broad with an intricate Celtic tattoo circling his right arm. He keeps his scalp trimmed down to an austere number one that is softened by an ever-present grin. Aside from the constant smile, everything about him, from his wide fingers to his heavy-set frame, suggests he is a strong and capable individual.

'I guess ours is a strange relationship but not that much stranger than many others. It only stands out as being different because the three of us live together. If Brenda and I were having an affair behind Andrew's back, people would think we were normal. Because I live with them, and we all know what we do together, it's looked on as being wrong.'

He chuckles and asks, 'Doesn't that say something about the value our society places on honesty in relationships?'

Waving the question aside, momentarily losing his constant smile, he says, 'Sex doesn't always have to be about love. Take a look around any swing party and you'll see that's true. Even in regular nightclubs and bars, where people are clumsily trying to get off with each other, they're not after sex because they love people. They're after sex because they're after sex. Sex is about having fun and doing things you enjoy. I know married couples who are supposedly in love and they treat sex as an occasional chore at the end of the day before they go to sleep. Sex is seldom about love. Sex is only ever about sex. Brenda's a very good friend. Andrew is a good friend too. Living with them makes our arrangement easier for all three of us. But I don't think I love either of them. I certainly don't love Andrew. I don't think either of them loves me. We're just good friends who have an open and honest relationship. We're good friends who have sex together.'

Charlie drives the car back home. Andrew and Brenda remain in the back seat, still touching each other and continuing to play. The sound of their enjoyment carries easily over the late-night radio station flowing from the car's speakers. Charlie makes a joke about stopping at a dogging spot and Brenda tells him to fuck off.

Brenda: 'We've talked about dogging, but I don't think that really appeals to me. Call me a prude but I think there's something tacky about getting banged across the bonnet of your car by a group of strangers in Tesco's car park. Also, I'm not into the whole chav fashion statement and, from what I've heard, a lot of doggers go for that sort of look.'

The banter between the three of them is filled with obvious affection and humour. Andrew suggests that Brenda might enjoy dogging if she could use the hood ornament from his

Jaguar as a butt-plug. Brenda asks him if he would like to have the hood ornament used on him as a butt-plug. Charlie winces and says it's fortunate Andrew no longer drives a Mercedes.

But all of this light-hearted teasing is tempered by the anticipation of something good that is still to come. Andrew has a hand at the top of Brenda's thigh, his fingers slipping close to the split of her wet and sensitive sex. Brenda perpetually shifts position so she can touch the back of Charlie's head and include him in the exchange even though he is driving. Charlie tries diligently to keep his focus on the road but, as every comment he makes is loaded with sexual innuendo, it is obvious that his concentration is not devoted solely to a safe journey along the motorway.

Andrew: 'Swing parties are good. Our occasional private time with other couples is also good. But great sex comes *after* those encounters.'

Brenda: 'It's almost as though the parties are like foreplay. Even though you can have full sex with two or three people. Even though you can come and come again at a party. When you get back home, and you're with the person you love, that's when the good sex becomes magnificent.'

Charlie: 'I don't understand why there should be a difference. But there is. The sex at the parties is fantastic for all of us. But the sex after the parties is always better. I don't know why but all three of us come harder and more forcefully when we play after a party. And, because we all know that we come harder after a party, we always make the effort to have that final get-together before crashing out for the night.'

Brenda: 'After a party, I find myself thinking about everything that we've done. I remember all the different guys I've been with, and all the different women. I close my eyes and see Andrew and Charlie with other women and it heightens my arousal. I think about all the sexy things we've done, seen and enjoyed, and it just makes the whole experience mind blowing.'

Andrew: 'It's just so much better. I don't know if it's because I've already come two or three times by that point, so I've built up the necessary longevity. Or if it's because I'm more sensitive. Or if I'm just more aware of all the eroticism that's been happening around me. But the sex after the party is the best ever. That has to be the main reason why we go.'

It's close to two in the morning by the time Charlie gets the three of them back home. They are all physically tired and mentally drained when they stumble inside. But none of them sleeps until two and a half hours later. And, by then, they are all truly satisfied.

Deborah

'... being intimate with a wide circle of friends.'

'I'm not a swinger,' Deborah says flatly. She is a pretty woman in her mid to late twenties. Ash-blonde hair falls to the small of her back. Her build is slender and willowy and shown off to great effect by her choice of clothes. The gypsy skirt, and a lacy top with dripping cuffs, suggests an interest in all things new age but she has already assured me she is a practising Catholic. Considering her home address is in Ireland, and she speaks with the dulcet brogue of that country, this final revelation does not come as a great surprise. 'I'm not a swinger,' she repeats, emphasising the point. And, so there is no misunderstanding, she adds, 'I just like doing this for my friends.' With that explanation given, she continues to masturbate Mike.

Educated in the restrictive atmosphere of an all-girls school and taught by nuns, Deborah believes her habit is an act of rebellion against a strict and oppressive upbringing. 'Convent educations are unnatural and unhealthy,' she says knowingly. 'The girls I went to school with either became frigid, neurotic or sluts. I think I'm the only one who found any middle ground.'

She wraps her hand tight around Mike's erection, squeezing to trap blood into the end of his length. The foreskin has already peeled back from his glans and turned a dark flushed purple. Smiling, Deborah loosens her grip and slides her palm over and along the shaft.

A crucifix adorns one wall. An illuminated reproduction of Christ sits on top of the dusty TV set. Aside from those two accoutrements, her flat is unremarkable and almost spartan in its simple furnishings. Plain carpets cover the floor and the wallpaper is so bland it is designed to be instantly forgettable. But Deborah compensates for the lack of homely comforts with her constant chatter and beguiling charm.

'More than a couple of the girls were into each other, which always creeped me out. I was young and very naive at the time. There was no sex education at St Mary's other than what we learnt from rumours and guesswork. But I knew that girls with girls wasn't normal. Girls with boys was normal and that was what I wanted.'

She grins at Mike, pushing him back in his seat and working her hand more quickly up and down. A pearl of pre-come wells in the eye of his penis. The veins along his erection stand bold and blue against the pallid flesh. He reaches from his position beside her to place a hand against Deborah's breast but she slaps it away with one quick, almost vicious, movement. Unperturbed, Mike lets the hand fall back to his side and allows her to continue.

'I got invited to my first school disco when I was sixteen,' she recalls. 'The brother of one of my friends from St Mary's made the invitation. Because it was a chance to socialise with boys, I leapt at the chance. The convent had done a good job of keeping me away from that sort of thing but it was inevitable it would happen one day. I was a very curious child.' Her smile is almost hidden as she turns her head, as though she is fearful of revealing a secret aspect of the curious child she is talking about.

The school disco she mentioned was the scene of Deborah's first sexual encounter. She was as curious about the boys as they were about her and it did not take long before she was outside with one of them and holding his erection in her hand. The excitement of discovering she could arouse her peers was surpassed by the pleasure of learning she could use this asset to make herself popular. After pulling him to a brisk climax, she found a small queue of boys had formed and they were all expecting her to provide a similar service. Deborah happily obliged.

'The idea of doing more with them did cross my mind,' she admits. 'But I never did. After such a strict convent education, I couldn't. I'd have been damned for all eternity. But I did enjoy pulling them off. There's no other sensation like it in the world. When you hold an erection in your hand, feel the life pulsing inside, and then you bring it to climax ...' She shakes her head, smiles bashfully as she blushes, and her voice trails off as though she can't find words to explain the phenomenon. 'There's no other sensation like it,' she concludes eventually.

The experience left her surprisingly satisfied, and with a penchant to continue handling erections. 'I stayed in touch with some of the boys from the party. The village where we lived was fairly small so it wasn't difficult to meet up with them again. But a lot of them soon grew tiresome. Some boys are surprisingly demanding. I've kept in touch with a few but too many of them think, because you've had their erection in your hand, you'll let it go everywhere else in your body.'

Before continuing, Deborah turns her attention back to Mike. Her hand glides quickly up and down his shaft. She varies her actions so that one moment she is working him fast, and then she is treating him to long leisurely strokes. Occasionally, she twists her wrist as she tugs on him, adding another variation to his pleasure. Every now and again, she pulls tight and leaves his exposed glans to pulse for an instant before carrying on. All the time she whispers words of praise into his ear, assuring him his penis is one of the most exciting she has ever seen and telling him that his prowess as a lover must be incredible.

Finally, she wrings the climax from him and Mike ejaculates.

Deborah releases a long, satisfied sigh as she milks the last drop of semen from the end of his glans. Her hands tremble as she gives him a chaste kiss on the cheek and then passes him a box of tissues.

Satisfied, Mike thanks her, and invites her to join him at the pub. When she declines, he promises to see her in the morning for their regular commute to work.

As Mike leaves, Dave and Vincent appear in the doorway and they enter together. They join Deborah in her lounge and sit on either side of her. Both men wear wedding rings and it is rumoured that Dave's wife is seriously unhappy about him visiting Deborah. However, no one mentions this situation as she unzips one, then the other, and proceeds to masturbate them simultaneously.

'I don't understand why so many people have a problem with my doing this for friends,' Deborah says. 'But, to hear people talk, you'd think I was committing war crimes.'

It is difficult to know whether Deborah is referring to the offended wives and girlfriends of those men who currently call on her, or the previous boyfriend she had briefly spoken about before Mike arrived. She claims they all act like injured parties and maintains their outrage is facile and unjustified.

The wife of one of Deborah's friends has recently subjected her to a campaign of menacing phone calls. Someone else (or possibly the same woman) has damaged Deborah's Fiat Panda and painted unflattering graffiti on the front door of her home. The sly attacks have started to taper off but the cruelty behind them left a mark that still causes Deborah some unhappiness.

'The woman has issues,' she explains with forced patience. She doesn't look at Dave when she says this. Her gaze is fixed on Vincent while both her hands work with an even and unbroken tempo. 'But there are a lot of people with issues. My last boyfriend wasn't too keen on the arrangement I had with my male friends. That was what brought our relationship to such an abrupt end.'

The relationship ended when Deborah's boyfriend returned home from work and found her masturbating Jason. Jason treated the situation with such equanimity that Deborah's boyfriend initially felt his anger must be misplaced and it is easy to understand that response. Every male visitor to Deborah's flat treats her welcome as natural and acceptable. They enter Deborah's room and receive a wrist job. She chats naturally and easily as she masturbates her friends, and can hold an asexual conversation with one man while wanking two others. She is so uninhibited and frank about what she is doing that reactions of surprise or upset seem totally out of place.

Consequently, it was only after Jason had left that Deborah's boyfriend finally voiced his reservations. 'You shouldn't be doing that for other men.'

'Why not? I've always done it.'

'You're going out with me now. I don't want you doing that for other men.'

'But it's only like shaking hands with them.'

'If it was only their hands you were shaking, there wouldn't be a problem.'

His anger then became apparent and the conversation reached an impasse. He wasn't going to have a girlfriend who wanked every man who entered her flat. And she wasn't going to have a boyfriend who dictated what she could and couldn't do with her closest friends.

'Not that I miss having a boyfriend,' Deborah remarks. She releases her hold on Dave and Vincent and ticks off the list of benefits on her glistening fingers. 'I've got Mike to give me a lift to and from work. Vincent here helps me with electrical problems. Terry is a plumber and Dave is always able to help me when my PC breaks down. When you've got a good network of friends, you don't need to have some man hanging around the place demanding cooking, fucking and a tidy home.'

With that said, she resumes her grip on both men and continues to stroke them back and forth. She also adds that, despite what people may think, she is not a swinger. 'Swinging is about being promiscuous,' she explains. 'And I don't think what I do is promiscuous. I'm just being intimate with a wide circle of friends.'

Dave clutches his thigh and stiffens against the settee. Vincent's smile is broad.

Deborah's hands work faster as she becomes more animated in her conversation. 'Swinging suggests people who are involved in open relationships. And I'm not involved in any relationship. I don't go to orgies. I'm nobody's wife, so it's not like I can have a husband swap me for the evening.' She glances poignantly at Dave and adds, 'Although I understand swingers are honest with their partners. And I must admit I'm never comfortable doing this for married men who keep it secret from their wives.'

Dave has been straining to stave off his climax. His efforts have involved rolling his eyes, balling his hands into fists and punching his thigh. But it only takes one stern glance from Deborah and it is apparent that his need to ejaculate is no longer an overwhelming force. His length wilts in her hand.

'I'm not saying anything against swinging,' Deborah continues. 'And, if people want to swing, I say let them do it. I'm just trying to say that it's not something I would ever do.'

And, although Deborah remains adamant that she is not a swinger, her argument is reminiscent of those smokers who maintain they are not addicted to their nicotine and could give up the weed tomorrow if they wished. She offers an explanation for her pedantic terminology when the subject moves on to religion. 'That's why I couldn't be a swinger,' she explains. 'If I had to go to confession and admit I'd been having sexual relationships with so many men, I'd die from the shame. Because what I do has nothing to do with sex . . .' She pauses, holding her right hand still on Vincent while pulling her left vigorously and repeatedly on Dave.

Vincent is struggling not to ejaculate. Clearly familiar with Deborah's rules, he keeps his hands by his sides and makes no attempt to touch her. Dave's erection had been waning but, with a few brisk tugs from Deborah, he is solid again and looks like a man hurtling to the brink of climax.

Deborah smiles and continues, both her hands once again working at the same leisurely pace. 'Because what I do has nothing to do with sex, I don't need to go to church and confess what I've been doing. All I'm doing is welcoming friends into my home. Confessing that to a priest would be silly.'

Dave comes first. Vincent ejaculates shortly after him. Deborah shivers noticeably, and thanks them both with a chaste peck. She leaves the box of tissues between them and then goes to the bathroom to wash her hands. While she is still drying the antibacterial handwash from her fingers, she asks if anyone would like a tea or a coffee.

None of which addresses the question of whether Deborah is correct when she says she is not a swinger, or if she is simply protecting herself with wordplay. Within the space of an hour, she has masturbated three men to the point of climax and it has been obvious that she has gleaned enjoyment from each ejaculation. The interaction is certainly sexual and, considering she has many partners, it is not unkind to describe her as promiscuous. But Deborah will not accept that she is part of the swinging community.

In her own words: 'I have a nice social circle of male friends and we help each other out. It's not swinging. It's simply a network of friends. It's a shame people want to put silly labels on everything and won't accept that we're all just giving each other a hand.'

Glen & Susan and Moira & Stephen
'What do you suppose our partners are up to?'

Stephen and Susan lie on top of the bed together. Their elbows rest on pillows so they can talk and casually caress each other's body. Both wear wedding rings and nothing else. They have been acquainted for less than an hour.

'You're comfortable with this?' Stephen asks.

Susan nods. 'You?'

'Oh! Yes.'

His eager smile and her encouraging touch remove the need for awkward conversation. His lips brush against hers. She pulls him closer: her fingers explore his broad chest, his toned stomach and then the thatch of curls that trails down to his groin. He finds her breast with one hand, and the other goes behind her back, encouraging their embrace to become closer. Their bodies connect and the pair enjoy a moment of blissful discovery as each is able to mould themselves against a previously unexplored partner.

Stephen can feel his erection pressing against Susan's pierced belly button. The ring of metal – something he is not used to encountering – chills his broiling flesh.

Susan is aware of the unfamiliar weight, shape and warmth of his hardness. She notices the scratch of her pubic curls as they scour against his thigh.

Both are attuned to every detail, thrilled by the moment and basking in the new sensations. Although the embrace is comparatively chaste, when they finally pull apart they are panting with obvious sexual hunger.

'You're a good kisser.'

'I do other things better.'

The remark is followed by a suggestive smile that has them giggling.

'What do you suppose our partners are up to?'

'Pretty much the same as us, I'd guess.'

'What do you suppose our partners are up to?'

'At a guess, I'd say pretty much the same as us.'

The comment sparks a knowing chuckle. Glen and Moira are in an adjacent bedroom and, although neither has yet removed their clothes, this does not present a barrier to their intimacy. Moira lies on the bed, her skirt hitched above her waist, while Glen kneels with his head between her legs. He slurps noisily at her sex, chasing his tongue against the shape of her labia and occasionally teasing between her warm wet lips. His hands rest lightly on her thighs and he savours the perfume of her pussy with obvious appreciation. Because Moira has shaved herself free from pubic hair, Glen is able to glide his tongue smoothly over her flesh before delving back between the split of her labia.

Like Stephen and Susan, Glen and Moira have known each other for less than an hour.

And the evening is going exactly as the foursome have planned.

Prior to the couples departing for the bedrooms, the conversation had been stilted. The etiquette at an initial meeting between swinging couples is often awkward, as everyone tries to accommodate the others' limits without transgressing their own personal boundaries.

Stephen and Moira have been swinging on a monthly basis for the last three years. It is one of the self-imposed rules of their recreational sex that they will never swing with the same couple more than three times.

Glen and Susan have been swinging for less than a year and, ideally, would like to meet a couple with whom they can share a regular swapping relationship. They know that Stephen and Moira are not looking for the same sort of arrangement, but they found their advertisement appealing and decided to enjoy a deliberately casual fling while continuing to look for their ideal.

The two couples met through an internet site for swingers. Initial contact was made a week earlier and, after an exchange of photographs and a brief meeting in a local pub, the four gathered for the evening at Glen and Susan's. After agreeing the night would progress as they had initially planned, Glen suggested Moira should join him in the privacy of the bedroom. Susan asked Stephen if he would like to accompany her to the spare room.

The kiss turns into an exploration. Susan's lips slip from Stephen's mouth, move over his chin and then down to his throat. He keeps his hands on her body – never losing contact with her warm soft skin – and allowing his grip to trail from her buttocks, over her hips and up to her waist. Her fringe brushes his chest as her kisses move lower. His upturned hands find Susan's breasts and he is not surprised to discover that her nipples are rigid. Catching the hard flesh between his fingertips, he gently squeezes.

Susan moans but her sigh is drowned out by the joyous cry from the adjacent bedroom. Moira's voice, dripping with arousal, begs for more. Her tone is so frantic and shrill it is obvious that she doesn't need too much more to be satisfied.

'Glen's very good,' Susan explains.

Stephen laughs. 'And Moira's a noisy bitch when she's enjoying herself. Do you think they're having more fun than we are?'

Her mouth hovers over the end of his erection. Each time she breathes out, a sultry breeze whispers against the swollen tip.

Slowly, she shakes her head. 'Glen's great at cunnilingus,' Susan explains. 'And I love it when he goes down on me. But I also love it when I'm with someone who does foreplay differently. I like the variety.'

Nodding his understanding, Stephen pulls Susan closer again. His fingers slip over the curves of her body and glide easily to the centre of her sex. His touch is light but commanding. When he strokes the wet split of her labia, she shivers. His fingers move slowly around the sensitive flesh, brushing over her clitoris, teasing the length of the lips, before eventually easing into her hole.

They both sigh. And Moira's shrill cry carries easily through the wall.

Glen rides Moira brusquely from behind. Each time he thrusts into her, the bed creaks from the force and she groans with obvious pleasure. They have still not bothered to undress, having only moved clothes aside to help them get closer to satisfying their immediate desires. Glen's erection protrudes from the open fly of his pants. Moira's skirt has been lifted over her waist and her thong has been pulled to one side. The fact that they remain fully clothed is a testament to their urgent need for each other.

'God! Yes!' Moira screams.

Glen chuckles and pushes deeper and harder. Her velvety wetness encircles his erection. Her sex makes a greedy slurping sound around his shaft each time he plunges inside. Moira is exceptionally loud with each response; her cries come with greater urgency as her climax nears. Glen holds her by the hips, pulling her back to him each time he thrusts forwards. The wetness of her sex has already been sufficient to trickle past the base of his condom to chill his taut sac. She clutches her muscles tight around him and they both groan with mounting satisfaction. Their bodies bang together with greater speed and more fury, as they each strive to take the other to orgasm before enjoying their own release.

Glen is panting; Moira grunts. And, when the orgasms come, they both groan with ecstasy.

'For me,' Stephen admits, 'the thrill of swinging comes from a lot of things. If I was trying to be all laddish, I'd say it's about getting to lay lots of different women. But that's not even half the truth. Moira and I go for a full swap and, from experience, we've found it works best if we're in different rooms. Same-room sex is a bit too tacky for our tastes, and it's very distracting. When we each pair off to a separate bedroom, I get my pleasure with another woman; Moira gets her pleasure with another man; and then we each get the additional pleasure of imagining what the other has been doing. The final pleasure comes the following day when we're able to tell each other exactly what we were up to.'

In his early forties, Stephen is not a particularly handsome man but his constant smile makes his appearance engaging. His muscles are toned from a weekly visit to the gym and he has sufficient confidence in his body to hold himself proud when he is naked.

'It's all about being erotic,' he explains. 'Moira gets to feel more erotic because there are men appraising her, showing sexual interest in her, and proving that they find her arousing. I'm seeing evidence that my wife is as desirable as I've always maintained and it's that additional appreciation that adds to our sex life.'

Now that Glen has come, Moira has removed his trousers so she can more easily suck life back into his limp cock. He is lying across the bed, his face buried under the folds of her skirt. Her sex, still wet, smothers his mouth and nostrils. Her thighs squash against his ears and she rubs herself lightly against his nose as he laps at her. The smooth flesh of her freshly shaved pussy is oily from perspiration and her copious musk.

'Make it go hard,' she complains.

Although her words come out harshly he can tell her impatience is mingled with humour.

'It's getting hard,' he says and chuckles.

He darts his tongue against the folds of her labia. The skin tastes of salted feminine musk and the latex of the condom he wore. After the vigorous session of sex they have just enjoyed, his penis feels exquisitely sensitive, yet he won't allow himself to remain flaccid. Moira is a desirable woman and, although they have both climaxed, he wants to enjoy that pleasure a few more times before the night is over. Tracing his tongue against her super-smooth sex lips, willing the stiffness to return to his penis, he tries to imagine what Stephen and Susan are doing in the adjacent room.

Susan is close to orgasm and Stephen has yet to slide his erection inside her. After kissing her bare body, he treats her to a sensuous massage that slowly grows more intimate. He has stroked her nipples until they stand rigid, then suckled against them while he slips his fingers against her sex. When Susan makes an attempt to reciprocate his caresses, he carefully moves her hands away and insists she lie still as he explores her. His fingers move deftly over her clitoris. Occasionally, he dares to tease inside her sex. Eventually, while he is stroking and she is panting, Stephen slides his finger inside her anus. Susan stiffens on the bed and then relaxes. Her breathing has deepened to a soft and satisfied sigh.

Keeping his hand cupped over her bottom, holding the finger inside and wriggling it gently against the delicate tissue within her anus, he moves his lips close to her ear and asks, 'How far do you want to go this evening?'

'I'm prepared to go all the way,' she says laughing. 'Or did you want to go further?'

He wriggles his finger until she stops laughing and begins to sigh again. As he slips it gently backwards and forwards, allowing the knuckle to ease past the muscle of her sphincter before pushing back inside, he says, 'I wanted to take you in all three holes before the night was over. How does that idea sound to you?'

Susan draws a deep breath. She shivers with anticipation. 'I think I could enjoy that.' Her cheeks are red with embarrassment and pleasure. 'I'm sure I could enjoy that,' she admits. 'But you'll need to use a little more lubricant if you're going to start where your finger is.'

Nodding, Stephen reaches for the tube of KY Jelly that sits on the bedside cabinet. He smears large dollops over his fingers before sliding a second into Susan's welcoming rectum.

As soon as Glen is hard, Moira rolls the condom over his erection and straddles him. She has opened her top to reveal her breasts and he fondles her with hungry appreciation. Clearly eager for satisfaction, Moira fingers her clitoris while she levers herself up and down his erection. With sharp, demanding gasps, she tells him how to squeeze and touch her breasts. Obligingly, Glen does as he is told. The effort of concentration he has employed in maintaining his erection is no longer needed as the arousal sweeps through him. Taking advantage of the rising excitement, he changes position and pushes Moira back to the bed.

She happily allows this manoeuvre and wraps her legs around his waist as he plunges into her. Once again, she begins to moan with sighs that are long and loud enough to travel through the walls. Her cries are barely stifled when Glen kisses her. They escalate to deafening proportions when he places his lips over one breast and suckles against her stiff nipple.

* * *

'We started swinging by accident,' Susan explains. 'We were on holiday with friends. All of us were feeling relaxed – probably a little tipsy – and things progressed from there. I can't remember if someone suggested strip poker, or if we'd gone for a late-night swim. Whatever the reason, I do remember that Glen and I ended up naked with this other couple and the natural thing seemed to be to fuck them.

'The following morning was a tense time for all four of us. I know it's a cliché to use the term "walking on eggshells" but that's what it felt like. I guess no one is ever sure how to act after their first swap. Especially when it's not been planned or discussed. Glen and me had both enjoyed our night with the other couple but neither of us wanted to be the first to admit as much.

'Even when we'd begun talking about it, and assured each other that there was no need for either of us to feel threatened, there were a couple of moments when we realised we needed to be careful. I asked Glen if the other woman had been a better kisser than me.' She smiles bashfully and adds, 'I've always been proud of my ability as a kisser.'

Glen refused to answer the question and said, if they were going to go with another couple, they couldn't ever compare lovers to each other.

'His argument made sense. We weren't going in search of better lovers. We were only trying to add to a sex life that was already pretty good. I agreed straight away, partly because it made sense, but mainly because Glen was suggesting that he wanted to swap again. After the previous evening, that was exactly what I wanted.'

Stephen stands in the bedroom doorway, watching Glen ride his wife.

The couple have their backs to him – Glen is taking her doggy-style over the edge of the bed. Moira is being buffeted repeatedly into the mattress, grunting with obvious approval and cresting another noisy climax. As he watches,

Stephen is not surprised to find his penis growing thick with arousal. He and Susan have just finished their first exploratory session of sex and he thought his strength was sapped. But seeing his wife being taken by the other man has stirred his arousal back to full force.

Susan appears beside him, grinning indulgently as she watches her husband with Stephen's wife. Like Stephen, Susan remains naked. Untroubled by her nudity, or the scene before them, she places a casual hand against his backside as they continue to admire the pair. The touch is familiar and intimate and yet strangely platonic.

'Are you watching us?' Moira gasps. She is glancing back over her shoulder. Her forehead shines with perspiration, and her hair and the remainder of her clothes are in complete disarray. The grin that falters on her lips is fighting for control of her expression with a pout of raw satisfaction. 'Are you two standing there watching us?'

Glen glances back over his shoulder and nods at Stephen and his wife.

'What are you?' he asks, grinning. 'A pair of perverts?'

They all laugh.

'Stephen and I were going to get a drink before we went back to bed,' Susan explains. She talks as though she has interrupted them during a conversation about books or movies. Listening to her matter-of-fact tone, it would be impossible to discern that her husband was having sex with another woman. Or that she has just experienced anal intercourse with a man she has known less than two hours. 'I wondered if you two fancied anything while we were down in the kitchen.'

Moira asks if she can have a glass of mineral water.

Glen clutches a fond hand against Moira's backside and says, 'I've got everything I need right here.'

Susan shakes her head and leads Stephen away as he blows a kiss to his wife. Moira winks at Stephen, and then throws herself back into the task of fucking Glen.

* * *

Over breakfast, the talk brushes easily over the intimacy of the previous night. The highs of the evening are revisited with coy phrases that lightly allude to their respective experiences. Stephen and Moira have spent the night with the couple but are now anxious to return home to Stephen's mother who has been baby-sitting for them throughout the night. However, because they have been enjoying the company of Glen and Susan, they happily accept the invitation to share breakfast with them before making their way home. There is none of the awkwardness or embarrassment that any of the foursome remembers from their first swinging experiences.

'Last night was fun,' Susan declares. She glances at Stephen as she makes the comment and the crease of her eyes makes him wonder if she is thinking about a particular aspect.

'A lot of fun,' Moira agrees.

Glen asks, 'Would you care to make it a regular arrangement?'

There's a moment's hesitation and then Stephen and Moira try to explain their rule about only seeing a couple three times. The discussion becomes momentarily serious as Glen and Susan try to sway them with the merits of having regular swinging partners, while Stephen and Moira persist in adhering to their self-imposed limit.

'With regular partners you don't have to worry about compatibility,' Glen argues. 'You've already discovered you're compatible.'

'But, with regular partners, there's a greater danger of our all becoming jealous of each other,' Moira returns. 'I'm sure none of us wants to risk that, do we?' She glances at Stephen for reassurance.

'There's the added bonus of a good friendship as well as a swinging relationship,' Susan argues.

'And the greater risk of an emotional commitment that we might not be able to handle,' Stephen adds solemnly.

The conversation moves round in circles, a serious and dry debate of emotions and responses that is the antithesis of their behaviour the previous evening. Where they had been disconnected from their regular partners, the couples are now touching each other for assurance and security. Where they had been interested only in physical pleasure and fun, now they discuss their lifestyles with a savvy intelligence and understanding.

Because the two couples are so fixed in their views, it is clear that neither will persuade the other to accept their opinion. But eventually, as Glen is pouring them all a third coffee while Susan clears away the plates, Stephen is able to call a suitable compromise.

'We've always tried to steer clear of seeing a couple more than three times,' he begins.

It's a rule they imposed on themselves for fear of growing too attached to others. Stephen and Moira value their love and don't wish to jeopardise it by having a regular relationship with another couple. Both worry that they are running a grave risk of endangering what they have with their swinging lifestyle. However, as long as the recreational sex continues to add to what they have, they are happy to enjoy the variety of different partners. But it is always done with the proviso that these other relationships never have a chance to develop further.

'It's one of our rules,' Stephen reminds them. 'But nothing is written in stone. You two clearly want a regular relationship with another couple and, while it's not something we've specifically desired, it is something we might consider.'

Moira studies him quietly as he says this, and it is clear that she has reservations about this statement.

As though he senses her disapproval, Stephen places a reassuring hand on hers as he continues talking to Glen and Susan. 'We'll give your suggestion some serious thought over the next month,' Stephen promises. 'And, the next time we see you two, if it's still something you desire, you can take another shot at convincing us that a regular partnership is what we all want.'

The comment provides hope for all four of them and leaves them to make plans for what they will do when they meet up in a month's time.

WHERE DO YOU SWING?

L ocation is an important part of swinging. Contact ads invariably state an explicit distinction between *travel* and *accommodate*, which is as vital to the final arrangement as age, gender, fantasy and sexual orientation. A vast number of couples report that their first experience of swinging occurred during the relaxed atmosphere of a holiday and this fact alone suggests that location is of paramount importance for swinging.

Holiday swinging – package tours specifically organised for open-minded adults – is available for those who want to take their swinging worldwide. Locations range around the globe from Adelaide to Zurich, stopping at most major tourist spots in between. Hedonism, the Jamaican resort, entertains approximately two thousand swingers each January. On the Cap d'Agde, a naturist resort on the French coast of the Mediterranean, swingers can enjoy their own private beach as well as a variety of swinging clubs in the local area. In America, through the organisational skills of the North American Swing Club Association (NASCA), large numbers of swingers often gather for weekend events at hotels booked exclusively for their use.

Swinging clubs in the UK are evenly distributed throughout the country, with the usual bias towards London, Manchester and other regional capitals. Styles vary from those that are laid out like nightclubs, or saunas, to those that are presented as themed hotels. While some couples eschew the controlled atmosphere of swinging clubs, there are many who enjoy the comfort of established rules and regulations, with staff to make sure that nothing untoward occurs. Those against swinging clubs point to poor standards of hygiene, expensive admission charges and complex rules about the consumption of alcohol on the premises.

As with all aspects of life, the truth is somewhere between these two extremes and usually depends on the individual participant's tastes and expectations. For every swinger who would never patronise a club, there is another who believes it is the best way to forge new acquaintances.

Swingers' parties occur throughout the country. It is difficult to assess the popularity of swingers' parties within the UK because so little facts are gathered on the subject. Swingers' parties do happen but participants are guarded about their involvement. Because the legality of this subject is difficult to define, and because media reaction to swinging is often extreme and unsympathetic, few of those involved have any good reason to come forward and admit their predilection. Announcements are usually made through a grapevine of established swingers – advertising often encourages unwanted interest from either the authorities or journalists in search of an easy exposé – and nominal fees are charged to cover the cost of supplying refreshments and other necessary overheads.

Parties can occur in any location from private homes to rented hotels or any other feasible resort that offers a degree of seclusion. Parties in the UK have been hosted in private mansions, off-season holiday camps and aboard large luxury yachts.

Parties fall into two categories defined as on-premises and off-premises. This differentiates those events where swingers can have sex at the party, and those where swingers can meet other swingers and then move on to have sex away from the party either at their own homes or local hotels.

Yet, despite the sexual nature of the parties, many swingers claim that the experience is more social than sexual. Participation is not mandatory and etiquette demands that no one is ever pressured to do anything. Usually, invitations are extended to couples only, although some exceptions are made for single females. Drug use is negligible and over-indulging in alcohol is severely frowned upon. The vast majority of partygoers practise safe sex.

In America, NASCA claim the average age of swingers lies between the ages of thirty and forty and state their members are mainly (but not exclusively) Caucasian and middle class. In the UK, the average age is believed to be fractionally higher, although, because they have an upper-age limit on membership, the UK organisation Fever Parties (www.feverparties.com), claim the average age of their members is 29.

The legality of swinging clubs and swingers' parties is a complicated subject, particularly in the UK. The descriptions of what comprises a brothel, the definition of living off immoral earnings and the far-reaching effects of the Disorderly Houses Act (1751) have all impacted to make this erstwhile private activity a matter of grave concern for the authorities.

Until there were amendments to the Sexual Offences Acts (2003), a brothel was described by case law as 'a place resorted to by persons of opposite sexes for the purpose of illicit intercourse'. This meant premises used by swingers (for swinging) could be classed as a brothel and charges could be brought against anyone hosting such an event. The 2003 amendment to this law now states, 'It is an offence for a person to keep, or to manage, or act or assist in the management of, a brothel to which people resort for practices involving prostitution . . .' This small distinction now means the organisers of swinging activities are less likely to face prosecution under that particular section of the Sexual Offences Act, although there are circumstances where it can still be applied.

If an admission fee is charged, the host is risking a charge of 'living off immoral earnings' unless an appropriate entertainment licence has been purchased. While entertainment licences are one way to circumvent this particular clause, despite their prohibitive cost, regular use of an establishment for swinging parties can lead to charges (again) under the Disorderly Houses Act (1751). Additionally, there is always the danger of being charged with the common law offence of corrupting public morals.

Dogging is the broad term used to cover those sexual activities that take place outdoors. The term has come to be associated with exhibitionist couples performing inside parked cars for groups of (mostly male) voyeurs. Activities in these encounters range from simply showing/observing to full participation and group sex.

There are several suggestions for the etymology of dogging. One version states the phrase was coined from the belief that voyeurs 'dog' courting couples in the hope of catching a glimpse of their intimacy. Another cites dogging as a contraction of 'walking the dog' because the phrase is often used in the context of an excuse for a late-night stroll by those voyeurs who frequent car parks and lovers' lanes. There is also an argument that the term has been chosen because outdoor sex is a natural practice for dogs: hence dogging refers to any sexual activity that takes place outdoors.

This broad range of suggestions indicates that no one truly knows how the term originated. The suggestion that voyeurs 'dog' courting couples doesn't take into account that those couples involved in this current trend are invariably there for the attention. Although the contraction from 'walking the dog' presents a pleasing image of sly

British voyeurism, the author has yet to encounter one reference from a dogging participant who mentions any genuine dog (i.e. *canis familiaris*) present at such activities. And, while it is true that dogs do take advantage of any outdoor location for their sexual practices, this is also true of every other creature including human beings.

Primarily a British pastime, dogging first made media headlines when former professional footballer Stan Collymore was exposed as a (then) active participant. His explanation of the etiquette involved, and the intricacies of establishing contact, has shaped the current beliefs of the dogging scene as it stands today.

Interior lights, left on in a vehicle, indicate a couple who want to be watched. Open windows suggest that voyeurs might be offered the opportunity to participate to some degree at the discretion of the exhibitionists. An open door is treated as an invitation to join in. Because of its clandestine nature, a lot of dogging occurs in poorly lit areas, and experienced voyeurs do carry torches. But, according to those participants interviewed in the process of making this book, reports of complicated flashlight signals are merely media exaggerations. In truth, the etiquette is nothing more than the standard common sense expected from any group of consenting adults. Activities are kept out of view of minors and the general public; disruption to the area is kept to a minimum; and the stated limitations of all parties are respected.

Lecturer Richard Byrne (Harper Adams University College), in his 2003 document *Setting the Boundaries, tackling Public Sex Environments in Country Parks*, indicated that the phenomena affects 60 per cent of the UK's country parks. Urban car parks are frequently used (multi-storey car parks and supermarket car parks) but these locations are more easily policed and this is an obvious deterrent for many doggers. The fame/notoriety of any popular urban dogging location will instantly spell its downfall as it is subjected to a greater level of police attention. The same is only true to a lesser degree for the country parks, as their remote locations do make policing them more difficult.

Legally, dogging is something of a grey area. There are laws to protect innocents from voyeurs and exhibitionists (Sexual Offences Act 2003, sections 66 to 68), but these are dependent on exposure being witnessed by unwilling parties, or voyeurism occurring without the consent of those being watched.

Police policies towards dogging vary throughout the country. Some authorities tackle the issue with a zero-tolerance approach, while others are less concerned with dogging between consenting adults and more interested in the associated crime that can occur as a result of the activity. Richard Byrne's document points out that country parks are often poorly policed and ideal locations for mugging, theft, rape etc. Police are aware of many unreported cases of these associated crimes where the victims make no complaint because they fear their involvement in dogging has put them on the wrong side of the law.

And yet, despite these dangers (or possibly because of them), dogging is escalating in popularity. Internet sites for doggers boast tens of thousands of members. Tabloids are replete with sensational stories of dogging on a daily basis. And contact magazines abound with details of how to become involved with local dogging activities.

Although there are no definitive statistics, it is widely held that doggers are predominantly white, generally middle class and aged between thirty and fifty.

Eve and Frank do fall into those broad categories, and have been kind enough to share details of their involvement in the UK's dogging scene.

Eve & Frank
'. . . twelve strangers in one night.'

E ve and Frank had been dogging before but this time Eve wanted more: a lot more.

Married for five years, and describing themselves as 'open-minded' rather than 'adventurous', their first time had been an accidental initiation. Driving home late from dinner with friends, Eve was a little tipsy and they were both sexually excited. Frank had the wheel and, as he drove, Eve sucked on his cock. Believing they had the quiet night roads to themselves, Eve made no attempt to disguise what she was doing. But, when they paused at traffic lights, a honking car horn made them realise they had been observed. Embarrassed, Frank stared straight ahead without acknowledging the other driver.

Eve was kneeling on the passenger seat with her head lowered over Frank's lap. She took his erection from her mouth for a moment and glanced behind herself at the car that had pulled alongside them. The driver had wound down his window and was giving Eve a cheerful and enthusiastic thumbs-up. His grin was massive and he kept nodding and moving his lips, as though trying to impart an important message.

Eve said afterwards the moment was a revelation. 'I was only wearing a short skirt and a thong. I had my backside up in the air, and this bloke must have seen everything. It was obvious he could see what we were doing and I'm sure the dirty bastard was asking if he could join in.'

Caught in the glare of the red traffic light, Eve stared wordlessly at the cheerful voyeur. The spell was only broken when the lights changed to green and Frank raced away from the scene at twice the legal speed limit. The couple collapsed into their respective seats, laughing madly at what had happened as Frank struggled to put distance between them and the car that had been alongside them. They had just about recovered from the shock of being 'caught' when they reached the A-road that would lead them back to their hometown.

'That was *horny*,' Eve said, giggling.

Frank baulked at her use of that particular word. '*Horny*? You found that exciting?'

'Didn't you?'

He nodded in the direction of an approaching junction. 'If you found that *horny*, perhaps you think we should be parking up there for an hour or two?'

Eve and Frank had been married for a little more than five years. She had retained the same petite figure he had found so attractive when they met at university and he still played enough Sunday-morning football to keep in a reasonably athletic condition. Five foot two, brunette and slender (but with large breasts), Eve was usually dwarfed by Frank's six-foot-three rugby-player physique.

To Eve's growing interest and astonishment, Frank told her that a right turn from the junction led to a notorious dogging spot. A colleague from his workplace had mentioned the site and, as Frank explained the sketchy details of what was reported to happen there, Eve grew more and more excited.

'I can't say why I found the idea so exciting,' she said afterwards. 'Maybe I was still aroused from what Frank and

I had been doing. I think I was quite excited by the fact that a stranger had been looking at my scantily clad backside while I'd been sucking Frank off. From that sort of start, it seemed only natural to go one step further. I told Frank I wanted to go there.'

'You want to go there?' Frank sounded amazed. 'Why?'

Eve reached for his lap and stroked him through his pants. 'I want people to watch us fuck,' she explained.

Frank indicated right and drove them towards the dogging site.

'It was terrifying,' Eve said afterwards, 'but in a good way. I don't know why people bother themselves with drugs. I'm not saying anything against drugs and drug users. If people want to fill their bodies full of chemicals, then let them get on with it. But I can't see the need for heroin or cocaine when you can get so high from a cocktail of sexual excitement and danger.'

Leaving the streetlights behind them, heading towards a relatively unfamiliar area, Frank drove the car towards the 'lovers' lane' his colleague had mentioned. Eve squirmed on the seat beside him, her knees constantly rubbing together, her buttocks perpetually gliding against the seat. The atmosphere inside the car was thick with anticipation.

Two miles down the road, Frank thought he had missed the turning. Glimpsing two flashlight beams, dancing in a forest of trees, Eve grabbed Frank's arm and told him they were almost there. The night outside was only broken by the car's headlights. Trees lined the road, hiding the moon and the stars. The flashlights they had seen disappeared as though they had never been there.

'Last chance to back out,' Frank warned her.

She shook her head and nodded towards the approaching junction. 'Unless you've changed your mind, let's do it.'

Frank drove them down the road.

'We saw a couple of cars as we drove down the lane but it was almost like everyone was hiding. We didn't see anyone outside, although it was so dark we would only have seen people if they'd been standing in the middle of the road trying to get run over. When we pulled into a space and stopped the engine, my heart was pounding. I heard the electronic click of all the doors being locked and I realised Frank had tripped the central locking. That made me feel a little bit safer but it also heightened my panic. He asked me what I wanted to do now and I thought about it for a full minute before I replied.'

Eve eased herself out of her thong. Their eyes were growing used to the darkness and Frank was amazed to see his wife removing her underwear. Her face was bruised by darkness, making it impossible to read if she was genuinely excited by the activity or simply unwilling to say nerves had got the better of her and she wanted to back out.

He remained silent as she knelt on the seat, with her backside held high in the air, and then bent over his lap. Removing his erection from his pants, she began to lick and lap at his stiffness.

'Do you think anyone's watching us?' Eve asked. There was so much tension in her voice Frank couldn't work out if that was what she wanted or what she feared. 'Do you think anyone's noticed what we're doing?'

A face loomed against the driver's side window. The yellow beam of a small torch shone into the car and Eve realised a stranger was watching as she sucked her husband's cock. The swollen purple end rested on her lower lip; she had her tongue against the slit; and she was being watched by a stranger.

'It was a truly horny moment,' she admitted.

The stranger's smile was apparent, although he was gesturing to the roof of the car.

Frank grasped the message he was trying to relay and said, 'He wants us to turn the interior light on. He wants to get a better view of you.'

'Do it,' Eve snapped.

Immediately, Frank flicked the overhead switch and there was a terse cheer of approval from outside. Aware that she had heard more than one voice, Eve glanced around and saw there were at least half a dozen strangers surrounding their car and grinning madly at her. The thrill of exhibitionism added fresh excitement to the moment. She knew there were men at her side of the car staring directly at the exposed lips of her sex and her unconcealed anus. Shocked by her own daring, she licked and sucked at Frank as though she was putting on a show.

'I wanted to look at the blokes standing outside the car. There were so many of them. I guessed most were excited, and I wanted to see if any were tugging themselves off. I didn't dare look though. I was excited but really scared. So I did everything I could to make my performance good for them.'

As she sucked on Frank's erection, Eve reached between her legs and began to play with her labia. The flesh was moist and warm to her touch. She splayed the lips of her sex and felt sure she could hear groans of approval from outside. While a part of her wanted to wind the window down so she could more clearly hear what was being said and see what was being done, she worried that might be seen as a level of encouragement she wasn't ready to give just yet.

'I came,' Eve admitted. 'I'd never done anything so daring in my entire life. But, with a dozen strangers watching me just fingering my pussy and sucking Frank's cock, I came. When Frank shot his load into my mouth, I came again while I was swallowing him. There was a cheer from outside the car and a couple of guys tapped on the windscreen to ask if they could have a go.'

Frank started the engine and drove quickly away.

They discussed the powerful excitement of what had happened and, as soon as they were home, they fucked until the early morning. Frank was high on the arousal of having seen his wife show herself off to so many men.

'It was like the mental version of Viagra,' he explained. 'Every time I thought about Eve showing her pussy to those guys outside the car window, my cock became instantly hard. Eve must have been thinking about something similar because, each time I got aroused, she was constantly wet for me. In the days after that first dogging session, whenever we fucked, it was like slipping into melted butter.'

Eve was exhilarated by the experience. And it was less than a week later before she told Frank, 'I want to do it again.'

For the second occasion, they were more prepared. Eve bought two boxes of condoms, a flashlight for the car, tissues and a new outfit. Frank gleaned as much about the protocol of dogging as he could from the internet, and they felt suitably prepared to enjoy another exciting night.

On the journey down, Eve stroked Frank's hardness through his pants and said, 'Tonight, I want to touch another man's cock.'

It was an exciting prospect and Frank drove more swiftly to their destination. The area still seemed dangerously unfamiliar as they drove along the unlit lovers' lane but, after the enjoyment they had received a week earlier, neither of them was as apprehensive. This time their anticipation was more powerful than their nerves and they were both looking forward to gaining more from the experience.

Frank switched the light on as soon as they parked. Eve had not bothered to wear underwear this evening and she unfastened her seatbelt so she could join Frank on his side of the car. He pushed his seat back so there was space for her, and allowed Eve to unzip his pants and withdraw his erection. While she was stroking the swollen end against herself, a bearded face appeared at the window. Eve grinned for him.

The stranger's eyes shone with obvious approval and he made a circling gesture with his hand, encouraging her to wind the window down. She glanced briefly at Frank, wondering if he was likely to raise any objections, and then did as the man asked. She wound the window all the way down, and the night's cool air flowed easily into the car.

Eve hadn't realised that her body was already lathered with perspiration from her excitement. It was true that she knew her sex was sopping with musky heat but she became aware of its intensity when the chill from outside flowed over her arms.

Straddling Frank, his erection deep inside her, Eve considered the man watching her.

He grinned broadly, stepped closer and asked, 'Can I touch?'

'If I can touch you,' Eve returned.

Frank moaned beneath her.

The stranger outside the car needed no further encouragement and unzipped his pants to reveal a passable erection. As Eve reached out of the window to touch him, he reached into the car and fondled her breasts through her blouse. The sensation of another man's hand against her breast was electrifying. Eve squeezed her pussy muscles tight around Frank's erection and took a firm hold of the stranger's cock. Frank touched her right breast while the stranger stroked her left.

Eve crested a giddy plateau of unimagined pleasure.

There were other voices outside the car. The beams from torches brushed over her face and glinted against her cleavage. Someone said she was a looker, and another said he wished he could have a piece of that. She even heard one voice suggest sticking around, 'in case the horny bitch wants more'.

Frank and the stranger managed to slip the blouse away from Eve's body. Because she wasn't wearing any underwear, her large breasts were revealed and both men were able to freely touch, stroke and caress her. Their hands moved easily over her bare flesh and the waves of arousal came with greater force. Eve knew the first orgasm of the night would be soon on her but she didn't want it to strike too quickly.

Leaning close to her husband, wishing she had thought to discuss all the practicalities before they had come out, she kissed him and whispered, 'I want to suck this guy's cock.'

'You filthy bitch,' Frank grunted.

She laughed. Frank had called her a filthy bitch many times in the course of their five-year marriage but he had never once used the term in a detrimental way. When he called her a filthy bitch in the car, she understood he was saying the idea excited him as much as it clearly excited her.

Eve tore a condom from the packet and rolled it over the stranger's erection. Bobbing her head awkwardly through the window, placing her lips around the sheathed shaft, she heard a whoop of muted cheers as she rode Frank and sucked the stranger.

His length filled her mouth. The chemical taste of the condom was vaguely sickening but her thoughts were fixed solely on the action of being taken by her husband while a stranger fondled her and shoved his erection into her mouth. She was distantly aware of the cheering voices, good-natured cajoling mixed with coarse comments of gruff approval. No one made any attempt to lower their voice as they appraised her 'nice tits' and several speculated on whether or not she was going to 'do a turn'.

The orgasm came in a sudden rush.

Frank had been holding back on his ejaculation and admitted, 'It had been a struggle not to come as soon as I saw her holding the first guy's cock.'

When Eve managed to suck the voyeur to orgasm, and felt his semen fill the condom in her mouth, she was struck by her own climactic response. Screaming with delight, and riding briskly up and down on Frank's length until he was unable to resist the urge, she pushed the stranger away and fell on to the passenger seat.

'Do you want more?' Frank asked. 'Or should I take you back home?'

He had wound the window back up but that didn't stop faces from clamouring against the windscreen and her passenger window. Eve realised she was sprawled on the seat, her bare breasts visible to anyone who wanted to look and her pussy open, exposed and leaking a white dribble of

Frank's come. The moment inspired a brief thrill of shame – she remembers the stench of sex and the feeling that she had done something wrong was intense and overwhelming – and she told him to take her home.

Yet, before they had made their way back to the A-road, she found herself wishing they had done more. By the time they returned home, Eve was telling Frank that, when they next went dogging, she wanted to be fucked by another man.

'It was another week that seemed to go on forever,' she explained. 'And I felt like I'd become a sort of Jekyll and Hyde character. By day I was going into the office, chatting ordinarily with the girls about what was happening on the soaps and getting on with my life. And by night Frank and I were fucking like bunnies, talking about what had happened at Longniddry Bents, and what we were going to do when we got back there. Our sex life had always been good and full of lots of passion but, once we discovered dogging, it just went ballistic.'

And yet, when they set off for their third visit, Eve decided she wanted to do something different. The Longniddry Bents car park becomes busy with doggers after 11.00 p.m., and Frank and Eve had planned their journey so they arrived half an hour after this unofficial opening time. As soon as they had parked, rather than switching the light on, they left their vehicle and went to find out what was happening in the other cars. East Lothian nights are not renowned for their warmth and they both wore dark hooded jackets and jeans. A handful of shadowy figures were already roaming through the darkness around them but the atmosphere was neither intimidating nor unsettling. A few muted torches danced in the periphery of their vision and Eve and Frank could see the glow of a car's interior light, almost hidden by half a dozen silhouettes. Holding hands, they went to investigate.

'Everything was deathly quiet until we were almost on top of them,' Eve said. 'The blokes who were watching were muttering encouraging stuff, but they were keeping their voices low. The only one not being particularly quiet was the woman in the car, but I could understand why she was making a lot of noise. I'd have been screaming like a banshee if I'd been getting spit-roasted.'

Forcing their way through the edges of the crowd, their unease quickly turning to excitement, Eve and Frank found themselves staring at a blonde on the back seat of a BMW. She was naked, save for a filmy top that was draped over her shoulders, and her backside was hanging out of the open car door. Inside the car, a half-naked man knelt in the rear seat, thrusting his cock in the blonde's face. A man stood outside the car, behind her, and Frank and Eve could see he was pounding a substantial erection between her legs. The blonde moaned each time he thrust forwards, and then lowered her head back to the cock she was sucking.

'This lass is up for it,' someone in the darkness whispered.

Eve turned to the man, intending to politely thank him for the observation, when she realised he was wanking as he spoke. His fist was wrapped tight around a modest erection, and his hand moved rapidly up and down.

Because she was wearing a hooded jacket and jeans, and because the country area was so dark, she realised he hadn't noticed she was female. With his attention fixed on the blonde in the BMW, Eve didn't think he would notice the detail unless she drew his attention to the fact.

And yet, even though she was standing amongst a crowd of unknown men, many of whom were freely masturbating themselves, Eve says that she didn't feel intimidated. 'We were all there for the same thing. We were all watching a gorgeous blonde sucking and fucking. And we were all getting off on it.'

The man pounding into the blonde groaned when he reached his climax. The blonde sighed, then pushed him aside and called, 'I want another one. I want another cock inside me.'

A couple of men moved closer to the car door cajoling each other, but neither made any attempt to meet the blonde's needs. Frank shuffled from one foot to the other and Eve immediately understood that he wanted to meet the blonde's request. Suddenly intrigued by the idea of watching her husband use another woman, desperate to find out how he would enjoy it and what the scenario would look like, she nudged him with her elbow and hissed, 'Go on.'

'Wouldn't you object?'

She rummaged through her pockets and pushed a sealed condom into his hand. It was all the encouragement he needed.

Frank stepped behind the woman as he pulled his zip down. Rolling the condom on to his erection, he teased the blonde's hole for a moment before she pushed hard against him. Her sex swallowed his entire length.

'I began to understand what Frank was getting from our dogging,' Eve explained. 'There was a thrill that I can't describe when I saw his cock going into the blonde. Part of it was pride: I could see she was enjoying it and I was thinking, "Of course she's enjoying it. Frank could make any woman enjoy that." But I think part of it was because we'd broken another taboo. You're not supposed to have sex with other people once you get married. You're certainly not supposed to *watch* your partner have sex with other people. Yet I was standing in the car park, watching him push his cock into this blonde, and I was really enjoying the experience.'

By the time Frank had finished, and the blonde was calling for another man, Eve was busy helping the man by her side masturbate. He had objected to her touch at first but, once she had pulled back the hood from her jacket and he had seen that she was undeniably female, he had allowed her to stroke his foreskin back and forth while he fondled her breasts. Although they were touching each other intimately, they were both fixedly watching activities in the back of the BMW.

'Until you've been there, you can't know what it's like. I was wanking this guy – Allan he said his name was – and Frank had just come back to me after fucking this unknown blonde. The smell of the trees was all around us, and Longniddry is close enough to the coast so you can smell the ozone off the sea. But I could smell her pussy on my husband and I could smell the pre-come leaking from Allan's cock. Guys were all around us wanking; the blonde was screaming for another cock; and I was on the verge of coming just from holding this stranger's dick in my hand.'

Frank suggested that Allan should see if he could assist the blonde in the BMW. After Allan had curtly thanked Eve for her help, the couple returned to their car and embraced each other with furious passion. Eve says they both thought about making love there and then but the evening had proved too intense for them to do that. Eve had not expected to watch (or enjoy) Frank having sex with another woman and they were both anxious to discuss their responses, reactions and plans for future encounters. Because they were getting so much from the dogging experiences, neither of them wanted to spoil it by going too far or exceeding the other's limitations.

And so they began the long drive home.

Frank noticed a pair of headlights in his rear-view mirror when they were back on the A1 but thought nothing of it. Because he and Eve were talking about what had happened, how they felt about it and what they should do next, Frank realised they had been driving for a full fifteen minutes before he realised the headlights were still behind them. It was at that point that the blue lights above the car began to flash and a brief siren sounded to warn them they were being pulled over by the police.

'We were both terrified when we got pulled over by the police,' Frank said. 'Neither of us knew what laws we'd broken but we'd been fucking strangers in a public car park and we were sure there had to be a law against it somewhere.

'The police officer examined the car, then asked us what we were doing out so late. According to the dashboard clock, it was close to one in the morning. We were both surprised that the time had sped past so quickly. I said we'd just been out for a drive and he said it seemed rather late. I said neither of us had felt much like sleeping and then he asked if we'd been drinking. Neither of us had, and if he'd thought otherwise I know he would have breathalysed me. But he did ask us where we'd been. I said Longniddry Bents and I could see a wave of understanding wash over his face. From the corner of my eye, I saw Eve turn crimson and I knew she'd seen the same expression. The police officer asked if there was anyone else up at the car park and I said we'd seen a couple of people there. He let us go after that, but I have to admit that moment with the police officer made my heart race faster than anything previously that night. I was imagining ruination; the end of my career; friends and family turning their backs on us; and all manner of shameful calamites.'

'But we still carried on dogging,' Eve said.

It was a month before they returned to the car park. The intervening weeks were interrupted by Eve's menstrual cycle and a lot of heated arguments about whether or not they were being foolish for pursuing such a risky diversion. Although the reasons not to go dogging made sense to both of them, the compulsion to return was impossible to ignore.

Consequently, after four weeks of debating the folly of their actions, they climbed into the car late one Saturday evening and headed off for Longniddry Bents. Theirs was the first car there that evening and Eve had made up her mind about exactly what she wanted.

'I wanted Frank to see me fucking twelve strangers in one night. I'd seen him fuck that blonde, and that had fuelled my fantasies for days and days after the event. He'd watched me wank Allan and suck that other guy the week before. But this time I wanted him to see me being fucked and I wanted it to be a big and unforgettable experience.'

Eve moved on to the back seat as soon as Frank had turned the interior light on. She wore a trenchcoat with nothing beneath and unfastened it so he could see she was naked. The lips of her sex were already glossy with arousal from the heat that had welled inside her as they drove down to the car park. Frank asked her if she was sure that she wanted this and Eve promised him that she had never wanted anything more. Their conversation was brought to an abrupt halt when a youthful face appeared at the window. Eve encouraged him to open the door while she continued to rub her fingers against her clitoris. The excitement of the moment was intense and powerful. She knew she could have squeezed an orgasm in an instant when she saw the stranger gratuitously admiring her. Struggling to keep her voice level, she asked, 'Do you want some of this?'

'Fuck. Yeah.'

'Bring as many friends as you can find and you can have the first go tonight,' she promised. Saying the words made her feel outrageous and almost brought her to the point of climax. She heard Frank groan in the seat in front of her and knew he was sharing the same pleasure.

The stranger disappeared from view but they heard him step away and then whistle loudly. Attuned to every detail, Eve heard the shuffle of footsteps approaching and she saw the muted glow of flashlights coming nearer. Her heartbeat raced and the flow of liquid warmth broiled between her thighs.

The footsteps stopped around the car and Eve could see pale faces pressing against the windows.

The first stranger – the one she had told to summon friends – pushed his head boldly into the car. 'My friends are here,' he said.

She beckoned him closer, holding out a condom.

He pulled down his pants, uncaring about the night's cold against his buttocks, and rolled the sheath over his erection.

Eve was aware of Frank watching intently as the stranger climbed into the car and positioned himself between her legs. She reached out to guide his cock inside her and then sighed as it pushed into her sex.

'It wouldn't have been a surprise if Frank and me had both come in that moment. I couldn't recall ever being so horny and I knew Frank was really getting off on what was happening. The young lad fucking me was barely in his twenties and he had a lot of stamina. I saw him moving his head down, as though he was going to kiss me, but I shook my head and said I just wanted fucking, not kissing. That didn't put him off and he lowered his head further and sucked on my right nipple while he continued to ride me. I came within moments and, as soon as he had pulled his cock out of me, I was calling for the next one.'

The orgasm was strong enough to leave Eve momentarily breathless. Her inner muscles convulsed and she realised she was enjoying a second climax when the first stranger erupted inside her. Shaken by the extreme responses, she wasn't sure if her body could cope with the excess of pleasure she had planned for the evening, but she had no intention of backing out now.

The second stranger took the condom offered by Frank and then pushed himself into Eve's dripping sex.

'I've spoken to other doggers who use lubrication. I can understand that no one wants things to go dry at the wrong moment but I didn't have any with me then and I didn't need it that night. I've never been wetter down there and that certainly helped me take the second one and the third one.'

More faces appeared outside the car and brought with them a clamour of muted noise. Eve was unable to see how many men were watching her, or waiting for their opportunity to slip between her legs, but she guessed it easily exceeded the dozen she had promised herself for the night. Gasping under the weight of a new lover, she simply accepted the fresh intrusion and basked in the delight of having sex with a stranger.

'Eve changed positions after fourth one,' Frank explained. 'She'd been on her back, taking it missionary-style, but I know she gets more pleasure from rear entry. When she turned around, then dangled her arse out of the back of the car, I understood she wanted more. I slid over from the front seat and put my face up against hers. Tears of joy had made her cheeks wet and the stink of sex was radiating from her in waves. Unable to stop myself, I kissed her and felt another orgasm shiver through her body.'

The memory of that kiss was probably Eve's last coherent thought of the evening. She knows that she had at least a dozen men that evening. The number of used condoms they found in the car's footwell easily went beyond that amount. But the majority of the night is now a hazy blur of pleasure and satisfaction.

'I was sore as hell for the week after,' she admitted. 'And I was walking like a cripple the following day. But it was more than worth it. I'd recommend the experience to anyone and I'm going to go back again very soon. It's addictive. And it's life-affirming. Being wanted by so many men – being used by so many strangers – it makes you feel alive and desirable. And the sexual satisfaction is stronger than anything you can imagine. I'd never thought of myself as an adrenaline junkie but I'm hooked on dogging. I'll definitely be back for more.'

Grace & Harry
'Last month, we hosted a Roman orgy. It went quite well ...'

The room is silent save for the murmur of a dozen or more mumbled conversations. Dark enough so that none of the couples can see the other guests properly, the tension in the air as strong as the tangs of their fifty different perfumes and colognes. From speakers that no one can see, the first haunting strains of Ravel's *Bolero* begin to whisper through the blackness. As the first reprise of the repeated melody ends, as the snare drums fractionally pick up their volume to enforce the music's hypnotic rhythm, a single spotlight illuminates the centre of the room.

For the first time since they have all gathered, the guests are allowed a shaded glimpse of each other. The dress code for the evening has been described as smart/casual. The gentlemen are uniformly attired in pressed slacks and shirts while their partners wear the latest styles of light summer wear to take advantage of the clement evening. Nervous smiles – some wary, others filled with expectation – glimmer from the shadows. Bracelets and jewellery jingle softly as hands are clutched in reassuring grips.

And everyone stares at the pair of near-naked women who have been illuminated in the centre of the room.

'The icebreaker is probably the single most important event for the success of a party,' Grace explains. Elegantly coiffured, and looking remarkably stylish in a tailored trouser suit, she speaks with an accent that has vague inflections of her European heritage. Her slender figure and confident posture make it obvious that she is a former ballet-dancer. Even sitting, her poise is that of someone blessed with infinite quantities of refinement. 'We know that most of our guests are fairly nervous when they arrive, and it's too much to expect anyone to make the first move. Often they've been travelling for a while; some of them don't know what's going to happen, so we usually organise something special, so that everyone's put at their ease.'

The slow crescendo of Ravel's *Bolero* continues to rise as the gathered couples get their first glimpse of the two dancers recruited to perform the icebreaker. An ebony-skinned girl – tall and striking – stands opposite an alabaster blonde. They are dressed in matching outfits – filmy lingerie that shows off their long naked legs and hugs their firm full breasts. Their dancing credentials are obvious from the enticing way they roll their hips as they glide around each other, to the bold assurance they invest in each erotic movement. As the spotlight brightens, the audience watch the pair circle in time to the music's commanding 3/4 beat. With well-practised synchronicity, they each reach out to stroke the other and their dance becomes more intimate.

'I leave Grace to organise the icebreakers,' Harry says. 'I leave her to organise pretty much everything.'

Harry is a managing director in his late fifties. A stocky man with steel-grey hair, he relaxes in an open-collared shirt and a rather fashionable off-the-peg suit from Burton's. He has been interested in the swinging lifestyle for most of his adult life but this was not a passion shared by his first wife. After the break-up of that relationship, Harry and his new partner, Grace, began to explore their mutual interest in swapping and swinging. Their marriage bridges a twenty-year age difference but neither seems troubled by this large disparity. Their obvious passion for hosting swingers' parties gives them a unity that is not always so apparent in other couples with more customary interests.

'Grace has a much better eye for what will work than I do. And she keeps in touch with a lot of dancers who are sympathetic towards swingers and swappers.'

The dancers' lingerie has been designed so it simply peels away from their bodies. The music grows louder. The pair continue to stalk each other. The ferocity of their eye contact is as relentless as the beat of the snare drum to which they are dancing. The matching negligees are first removed, revealing each woman in only her French knickers and bustiere. Hands rest against arms and hips. Tongues slide over glossy lips as though this is nothing more than the prelude to a kiss.

And the spotlight grows subtly brighter. Dim bulbs in the ceiling begin to glimmer, allowing the audience to discern shadowy figures around them. But, as the two dancers begin to kiss, no one is watching the other guests. Matching every movement to the *Bolero*'s beat, they each ease away the other's bustiere, and then become more intimate.

Mouths mash together as the pair kiss. Bared breasts are cupped, caressed and squeezed. Still moving in time to the swell of the *Bolero*, the dancers entwine their legs as their hips continue to roll. Gussets press against thighs; one woman sighs and the other woman moans; and then they tumble to the floor.

As the dark girl sucks at the breast of her blonde partner, murmurs of appreciation begin to travel around the room. Couples exchange opinions on the performance between themselves and their immediate neighbours. The atmosphere of anticipation remains in the air but the tension has now softened.

Grace and Harry walk surreptitiously through their party, handing out glasses of Champagne. With more than a hundred guests, it takes some time to serve them all but the *Bolero* is a lengthy piece of music and, because the content of the show is becoming more exciting, no one is in any great hurry to go elsewhere.

'It would be easier if we had a couple of waitresses,' Harry confides. 'But, unless they were into the lifestyle too, that would seriously complicate things.'

The dark-skinned girl peels the blonde's panties aside. She reveals a pale expanse of hairless flesh.

Someone in the audience gasps and the mutable atmosphere shifts to something that is almost electric. As the blonde's pussy is licked and lapped, as she writhes in tempo to the music, the audience's appreciation and anticipation become more obvious. At first it is difficult to tell if she is genuinely enjoying herself, or if her gestures are coincidental to the waltz-like rhythm.

The blonde eases herself from the other girl's kisses. After pushing the woman to the floor and kneeling between her legs, she eases her panties away and then buries her nose against the wet flesh.

The exchange continues: varying with each reprise of the haunting melody. After kneeling, squatting, suckling and lapping, they eventually lie in a 69 position. By the time the final refrain of the *Bolero* is playing, the pair are licking each other with furious hunger. Mirroring their movements to reflect the crash of cymbals and the discordant blare of trumpets, they push away to take their applause from the party of swingers and swappers.

'I try to do something different for each icebreaker,' Grace explains. 'But the *Bolero* is perennially popular. I don't know if it's something to do with Bo Derek in that movie *10* or if a lot of our guests were big fans of Torvill and Dean. Whatever the reason, I know that plenty of people ask if we can organise that same show for the next time they're going to visit.'

'After the icebreaker, I inform everyone that canapés are available in the dining room,' Harry explains. 'Grace is a fantastic hostess and she will go from one couple to another introducing them to others who she thinks they will fit in with. She's also an outrageous flirt –' he laughs '– and I think she spends the opening hour of the party deciding who she wants and whether or not she's going to have them.'

Smiling at her husband, Grace says nothing to confirm or disprove this hypothesis.

The party is already under way and Grace is confident it will be a success. Some small cliques are already gathering. A handful of couples approach the dancers, congratulating them on their performance and exchanging intimate kisses. While some do make their way to the dining room, more make their way to the pool and others go off to the designated playroom. Light jazz has replaced the theatrical styling of Ravel and the house is animated by the sounds of gay chatter and horn melodies.

'No one knows what to expect when they first come to one of our parties,' Harry says. 'But, by the time they're on their third or fourth party, I've heard people saying, "Oh! They're doing that this time! Great." Last month, we hosted a Roman orgy. It went quite well because togas are so practical for our purposes.'

'Different people come for different reasons,' Grace elaborates. 'Some only want to watch. Others want to do much more. The playroom is always a favourite place but I think that's because playrooms are so unique. Where else can a person go to bed with thirty other people at the same time?'

A sumptuously decorated table dominates the centre of the majestic dining room. A handful of couples peruse the food while others act as though they are alone. An oriental woman sits naked in one of the many captain's chairs that line the walls. She is petite with her skin pale gold in the room's muted light. Her jet-black locks glisten midnight blue from the shadows. Each time she draws a breath, it is released with a shudder that makes her small breasts tremble. Her mouth is open in a perfect 'O' of contentment.

A woman's head nuzzles between her spread legs. Undressed to reveal her filmy lingerie, the stringlike strap of her black bra cuts through the pagan tattoo on her shoulder. With obvious enthusiasm, she laps and sucks wetly.

Behind them, two men watch with smiles that threaten to burst. One strokes the buttocks of the kneeling woman. His hand creeps close to her sex and elicits a shiver. She turns to face him, her lips glossed and shining.

The oriental woman carefully reaches out to the woman and guides her face back to her sex. Acting with confidence and control, she gestures for both men to step towards her and then daringly rubs their erections through the front of their pants. None of the foursome seems to care that there are others walking close by as they all become acquainted. No one objects when the oriental woman releases one erection and then the other. It barely raises an eyebrow on the passers-by when she starts darting her tongue from one swollen glans to the other.

'By the time they're attending their second or third party, the majority of our guests know what they want from the evening,' Grace explains. 'A lot of married women crave the chance to experience sex with another woman. Just as many men want to see their wives doing that. Even kissing, with just a little naughty touching, can be exceptionally erotic when it's between two women. But it usually leads to more. I think that's one of the things that happens most often at our parties. Women get to fulfil that fantasy.'

By the side of the pool a man and a woman are kissing. His shirt is open and her hands rove over his bare chest. He has one hand on her backside and pulls her close to his body so she can feel the weight of his erection through his pants. There are naked swimmers splashing in the pool, their cheerful cries echoing hollowly from the surface of the water. But they go unnoticed by the pair who are kissing. The couple are even oblivious to their respective partners, who have slipped from the seats next to them and are heading towards the pool's changing rooms.

Another couple, obviously newcomers, hold hands and watch a man suckle against a woman's breast as she moans and sighs. They exchange a sly glance and then share their own passionate kiss.

'Obviously there are some rules,' Grace admits. 'But we try not to emphasise too much on "don't do this" and "don't do that". We find it more conducive to the party atmosphere to say: do have a good time; do respect other people's limitations; do everything you've ever wanted to do.'

'There are some things Grace and I don't particularly like,' Harry explains.

'Watersports has never struck me as being sexy,' Grace adds. She wrinkles her nose with disgust. 'And I can't understand the need for anal sex. But I know watersports happens in the pool changing rooms. And, if I went around watching every couple to see if they were having anal sex, I wouldn't have time to enjoy the party myself.'

In the pool changing room, a naked burly man lies on the tile floor. Above him, a Rubenesque woman wearing only stockings and heels pushes her sex over his face. Her buttocks are large and pale. Her cleft is covered by a lush forest of dense, dark curls. Excitement and anticipation have made her labia moist. As she squats, the lips of her pussy peel apart and reveal the rich, sopping pink of her arousal.

'Are you sure?' she breathes.

'Yes. Go on.'

'Is this *really* what you want?' Her voice is a tease. She wriggles her haunches closer, almost allowing the lowest curls of her sex to brush against his nose.

He is sporting an erection – unsheathed at the moment – and it's obvious he is enjoying the exasperation she has created. 'You know it's what I want,' he gasps.

'Do you want to taste it?'

He groans, and then lifts his head slightly. When his tongue glides against the sodden lips of her sex, they both shiver from the pleasure. Her sex is musky and rich with the flavour of arousal.

'Do you want to taste more?' she taunts. She sounds breathless, as though the experience is already pushing her to the brink of orgasm. 'Do you want to taste more?'

'God! Yes!'

She squats down, pushing her sex over his mouth. And she lets herself go. A golden shower of urine pours over the burly man's face. The warm liquid squirts into his eyes, up his nose and soaks his hair. His mouth is open so his tongue can squirm against her gaping sex. He spits, swallows and splutters, as he tries to pleasure her while basking in the joy of the scalding stream.

'We manage four or five parties a year,' Grace explains. 'Harry likes to have his themed events – the Roman orgies, the school discos, vicars and tarts – but I prefer to keep things less formalised. I think people are more able to do what they want without the restrictions of fancy dress. Not everyone comes to have sex. A lot of people simply enjoy being turned on by someone other than their regular partner. The laissez-faire style of my parties is more conducive to that sort of interaction.'

'Whichever style of party it is,' Harry continues, 'there are some things that always remain the same. Some wag always makes a balloon out of one of the condoms. Someone always has sex in the pool. We keep finding thongs and socks for the best part of a month after. And we always have too many people in the playroom.'

In the main lounge, three near-naked figures writhe together where the dancers put on their performance. They are oblivious to those around them, none of them aware that they are being absently watched.

One man lies on the floor with the woman straddling him. His erection is buried deep into her sex and, from the contortions of his face, it is obvious that he is struggling to stave off an impending orgasm. She is clearly showing no restraint. Her neck muscles strain and her cheeks have become flushed as another orgasm batters its way through her body. The man on top of her, the third party in this impromptu threesome, is also forcing his erection between her overstuffed sex lips. His sheathed shaft rubs against the first man's stiffness; the pair are struggling to adopt some unity in their rhythm as they ride in and out of the woman between them and it is obvious that their concentration is fixed on the moment.

Those around them occasionally glance in their direction. The sound of a loud groan or a startled expletive is always enough to call attention. But most of them are too busy touching, talking, kissing, laughing and exchanging smouldering glances to spare too much time watching the threesome.

Another couple are having sex on the stairs. Music from the lounge is just audible: an undercurrent to the animated conversations sounding through the rest of the house. Gasps and cries come from above them as the playroom becomes more populated. People continue to walk up and down the stairs, mumbling 'excuse me' and 'sorry to trouble you', as they pass the passionate couple.

He is unclothed save for his shirt. The discarded pants at the bottom of the stairs belong to him, as do the shoes and socks. They lie in a forgotten jumble with her knickers and one of her heels. She wears a short skirt that is pulled up to her waist exposing her bare thighs and open pussy. Her blouse is open, allowing her sumptuous breasts to spill free. She groans enthusiastically each time he plunges into her. Neither of them seems concerned that everyone else is making their way past them towards the playroom.

'We have the occasional spot of trouble,' Harry admits. 'But it's seldom serious. I think we've seen one fistfight in ten years of hosting our parties and that was just because one bloke was incredibly pissed and the other bloke was incredibly stupid. If any of our guests do have a difference of opinion, most of them simply agree to disagree and then walk away.'

'No one comes to our parties to fight,' Grace agrees. 'Swingers are laid-back in their attitudes to most things. Anyone who wants to watch their partner have sex with someone else has clearly got a well-adjusted grasp on their personal jealousy issues. That's not the sort of person who is going to turn abusive without any warning. I'm not saying swingers don't get jealous,' she adds quickly. 'For some people the jealousy is almost as much of an aphrodisiac as the party experience itself. I'm just saying that swingers have usually proved their ability to control their jealousy and make it work for them.' Laughing, she says, 'If anyone at our party really were the jealous type, their head would probably explode if they went into the playroom.'

Noise from the playroom is audible along the whole of the first floor. Few words can be discerned but it is obviously a sexual sound. Grunts, sighs and muffled exclamations are jumbled together in myriad layers of explosive pleasure. Closer to the playroom, the scents of clean perspiration and feral musk perfume the air. On entering the room, the first thing everyone notices is the mass of bodies joined together. The size of the bed – four doubles bound together at the corners – almost always goes unnoticed on a first impression. It is the sight of a dozen naked bodies, sliding freely together and gliding easily against each other, that catches the attention.

Erections, breasts, pussy lips and tongues are joined in countless variations of a familiar theme. Strange hands touch unfamiliar bodies. Kisses are exchanged as nipples are teased and cocks are stroked. Some fucking occurs in the centre of the bed: a sheathed length slipping in and out of a welcoming warmth; painted lips encircling a thick sheathed shaft. The woman at the centre of the bed is having one breast sucked, the other squeezed, and she has her tongue plastered against another woman's sex.

It would be impossible to describe every encounter on the bed. As the dozen bodies become twenty, fresh naked flesh brushing the sweat-slick skin that already resides there, it is apparent that the playroom is the place where most of the guests want to be.

The variety of body shapes, sizes and colours is as broad as the range of interactions. Cellulite, potbellies and stretch marks are sprawled beside and on top of aesthetic perfection. Long coltish limbs intertwine with knock-kneed legs. Slender manicured fingers squeeze plump and sagging breasts. No discrimination is made on the grounds of physical perfection or a lack thereof. Everyone is welcome in the playroom.

Not everyone is involved in a penetrative act. One woman gives oral to her husband while she receives it from another man. Two women lie in an unbreakable clinch, smiling for each other whenever they are touched or caressed by the others on the bed.

Even those who are spent continue to lie on the playroom's massive bed and enjoy the singular experience of being surrounded by so many naked lovers. The numbers continue to increase and it is only eventual thirst that drives them slowly from the room.

'The length of our parties varies but we've usually said goodnight to the last of the guests by around two or three in the morning. I make a point of asking newcomers what they're expecting out of the evening and then I try to organise it for them. If a couple tell me they just want to watch and meet people, I'll introduce them to guests who I know are show-offs. Occasionally, we have couples arrive where one is eager to participate and the other is obviously reluctant but that's never a big issue. No one ever pressures anyone to do anything they don't want – that *is* a rule – but, even if someone is there under duress from their partner, they're never forced to do anything.'

Harry agrees. 'The men at our parties are gallant and wouldn't approach a woman if she looked less than enthusiastic. The women at our parties are more interested in those men who want to be there. You can spot reluctance and unease a mile away and no one comes to our parties to find someone who doesn't want to be with them.'

Parting kisses and thanks are exchanged with names and numbers at the end of the evening. Most couples depart together and leave the party behind, although there are always some that share a car with the obvious intention of continuing their fun elsewhere. Alone, Harry and Grace retire to bed where they discuss the high points of the evening and the personal experiences they have each enjoyed.

Invariably, they make love before sleeping.

'I think every couple should visit at least one swingers' party,' Grace confides. With a knowing smile directed at her husband, she adds, 'But, if they really want to enjoy the experience, it has to be one of my affairs and not one of Harry's fancy-dress parties.'

Tony & Tanya and Lisa & Leonard
'A couple to her left are sighing in unison.'

Two couples sit in the foyer of the swingers' club and it is difficult to decide which man belongs with which woman. They chat affably together beneath the glow of sultry neon, laughing easily, and idly placing hands against the other's arms and legs.

Behind them, the window to the outside world is polarised and has darkened the pleasant dusk so the evening looks like it is threatened by an impending storm. But, inside the reception, the walls are a soothing green and the lights are dim enough to suggest a tranquil mood.

Tony has the build of a bricklayer, and the rugged countenance of someone who works outdoors. Leonard appears to be Tony's senior by at least five years but his complexion is characteristic of someone usually confined to an office with his face only illuminated by the glare of a PC screen.

The women between them are both dressed in short skirts, stockings and heels. Each wears her hair as though it has been freshly coiffured for this occasion. While their styles are clearly different – Tanya is going for an effect that is best described as obvious, while Lisa's apparel is slightly more conservative – they both look as though they have dressed to impress. Tanya is large-chested, with an infectious laugh that rings loudly around the clean and welcoming foyer. Lisa is slender and petite but she carries a smile that is as warm as the other woman's laughter.

The conversation touches on their mutual reasons for visiting this club and Tony is frank in his admission of what they want from the evening. 'We both want to get fucked,' he explains. 'Isn't that what everyone wants?'

Leonard and Lisa smile politely but neither speaks.

'I come here to suck cock,' Tanya confides. She shivers as she makes the admission and the tremor goes all the way through her ample body. She grins at Leonard and Lisa as she whispers, 'It's such a turn-on to take another man's dick in my mouth. I get *so* wet.'

'It's what you make it, isn't it?' Lisa comments sagely. Her voice has the soft lilt of a Welsh accent.

They all agree that this is true.

Before the conversation can continue, the young lady from the reception desk reappears and tells Tony and Tanya she has confirmed their membership and they can now go through to the main body of the club. She hands them a pair of locker keys and two large towels before wishing them a good evening inside.

Clearly excited, Tony thanks her, while Tanya promises Leonard and Lisa she will watch out for them. Handshakes and kisses are exchanged before Tony leads his wife through the double doors leading into the club.

The receptionist waits until the younger couple have left before asking Leonard and Lisa if she can help them.

Leonard flashes a joint membership card at the receptionist and says they will be going through in a moment. The receptionist glances at the main doors, as though she can still see the retreating figures of Tony and Tanya, and nods silent understanding.

* * *

In the changing rooms, Tony and Tanya chatter animatedly as they undress. Their walk from reception allowed them a brief glimpse at the first floor of the club and they are now both bristling with excitement and anticipation.

'Did you see those two lasses kissing in the pool?'

'I saw them. They looked hot.'

'Maybe it's a heated pool?'

'You daft bastard. I meant they look sexy, not sweaty.'

'I knew what you meant. I was just kidding.'

Tony glances around the changing room, calmly assessing the spartan décor. Small lockers face wooden benches. The floors and walls are beige tiles beneath a suspended ceiling and fluorescent lights. The effect is surprisingly bland and uninspiring. A tang of bleach lingers in the air. The fragrance is not particularly pleasant but it is faint enough to let him know the club is clean. The nuisance of that particular smell is forgotten as he catches the stronger scents of the chlorine used for the pool, then the fuller zest of Tanya's perfume, revealed as she removes her blouse and skirt.

He smiles, as he always smiles, when he sees her body exposed to him. The black straps of her bra and thong cut into her shoulders and her hips. She has been building up her tan over the summer months and the sun's rays have bronzed her flesh and darkened the Daffy Duck tattoo on her left buttock. Unable to stop himself, Tony places a large hand over Daffy Duck and gives his wife's rump an affectionate squeeze.

Tanya giggles and moves his hand away. 'Save it for inside the club.'

'We *are* inside the club,' he points out, making another grab for her.

'Properly inside the club,' she warns. 'I didn't come here to get a quick fuck in the changing rooms.'

Reluctantly, Tony stops making attempts to grope his wife and continues to remove his clothes. 'Is this what you were expecting?' he asks. When Tanya meets his gaze, he gestures towards the bays of the changing rooms that lead out through to the pool area. 'This place,' he clarifies. 'Is it what you thought it would be?'

This club is different to the others they have tried in the UK, with a pool dominating the central area of the ground floor. The other clubs they have visited were fashioned in the style of a nightclub, but someone has dared to be different with the layout for this one. A soft-drinks bar and sauna are also on the ground floor. Signs for upstairs indicate there are four or five playrooms above. But, although they only got a brief glimpse at the ground floor as they hurried to the changing rooms, they have noticed there are quite a few couples scattered around the sides of the pool.

By the time Tony has finished stripping and is folding his clothes into the locker, Tanya has still not answered his question. He glances at her – she has draped the towel around her large breasts and looks as though she is intending to visit the club's sauna first – and asks again, 'Is it what you thought it would be?'

She smiles and offers him her hand. 'Let's go and find out, shall we?'

Tony shakes his head, reaches inside the locker and produces two small miniature bottles of alcohol that he has brought with him. The swingers' club is unlicensed and the literature they received prior to attending has forewarned them that only soft drinks are on sale, although there is provision for swingers to bring their own alcohol and have it stored behind the bar. Not wanting to waste time with the trouble of storing drinks, Tony has just brought a couple of their favourite miniatures.

Tanya downs her Southern Comfort while Tony quickly swallows his Jack Daniels. He tucks the empty bottles back into the locker and then takes Tanya's hand. 'Now I'm ready,' he declares.

Together, they walk into the main body of the swing club.

* * *

'Do you just work here?' Lisa asks the receptionist. 'Or is this –' she waves a coy hand towards the main doors '– your kind of thing?'

The name badge above the receptionist's breast says her name is Kate. Kate explains that she knew the owners before they had set up the club in the town centre. They met when she responded to a classified advert they had placed for a bi-curious woman. Kate formed a close friendship with the husband and wife team behind the club and, when they told her they were looking for staff, she had left her job as an administrative assistant and taken on the role of receptionist. Smiling slyly at Lisa, she finishes her explanation with the words 'Why do you ask?'

Lisa blushes. 'I was wondering if I might get the chance to see you inside,' she manages.

Kate shakes her head. 'I've got to stay behind the desk,' she explains. 'But, if your husband doesn't mind waiting for us, you could join me here for a moment.'

Lisa is with her straight away. And, as Leonard remains in the comfortable seating of the foyer, he is able to watch his wife and the pretty receptionist kiss and touch. It crosses his mind that, if Kate was bi-curious when she first met the club's owners, she still seems eager to satisfy her curiosity. Her hands move to the back of Lisa's head, pulling her into a kiss that is passionate, long and torrid.

Although Lisa is usually reserved, she gives herself to the kiss with an urgency that she normally contains. Her hands explore Kate's body with avaricious haste. Curling one leg around the woman's hips, stroking inquisitive fingers against the swell of Kate's breasts, Lisa draws a deep breath as the rush of arousal sweeps through her.

Kate's hands move from the back of Lisa's head. She trails her fingers down the other woman's back before cupping her buttocks and making their embrace more sexual. As the pair grind their pelvises dryly together they both gasp as though the electricity of the moment has finally shocked them. Reluctantly, they step apart.

Kate's eyes shine with devilish excitement.

Lisa continues to blush – her smile is lascivious and hungry.

'My shift here finishes at ten,' Kate tells Lisa. She hands over a pair of locker keys and large fluffy towels. In a voice that sounds incredibly casual, she asks, 'Do you want me to come and find you if you're still in here then?'

'I think that would be fun,' Lisa whispers.

Leonard nods his approval and takes his wife's trembling hand as they finally make their way inside the club. As they step through the main doors, they hear someone cheerfully shout, 'Hi!'

'Hi!'

The simple greeting stops Tanya from making it to the sauna. A naked brunette is emerging from the pool, waving for her attention. The woman is slender, carrying the telltale paunch of recent motherhood, with breasts that only sag a little. Her nipples are tiny, almost without areolae, but they stand dark purple and erect against her pale skin. She wears a smile that is made appealing by a tinge of genuine warmth.

'I saw you coming in,' the brunette says as Tanya kneels down to meet her coming out of the pool. 'I simply loved those boots you were wearing. Are they Prada?'

Laughing, Tanya shakes her head. 'Versace,' she explains. 'They hurt like hell to walk but I think they look fantastic.'

'They made your legs look great,' the brunette says. She raises one hand, still dripping with pool water, and tentatively reaches for Tanya's calf.

Kneeling by the side of the pool has allowed Tanya's towel to fall open, exposing the fact that she is naked underneath. She knows that her sex, stomach and the underside of her breasts are possibly on display but, in this environment, that doesn't really matter. She can see an unspoken question in the brunette's glance and nods softly, silently giving permission for the woman to touch her leg.

Now the brunette is out of the water, Tanya can see she is completely naked. Her sex is free of pubic hair, with only a shadow of stubble darkening the flesh between the tops of her thighs. Raising her gaze to meet the brunette's eyes, she sees the familiar signs of excitement and expectation glistening in her smile.

'I do like great-looking legs on a woman,' the brunette admits. As she speaks, her slippery fingers stroke up from Tanya's calf to the back of her thigh.

Tanya shivers. Suddenly breathless, aroused and unsure if she wants to be excited in this way, she hesitates before responding to the caress.

'Aren't you looking to meet a woman here tonight?' the brunette asks. She delivers the question in an innocent voice that belies the fact her fingers are stroking small and delicate circles against the back of Tanya's thigh.

'I didn't come here looking to meet a woman,' Tanya admits. She thinks of saying that she came to suck cock. Instead, she reaches forwards, brushes a few stray hairs from the brunette's cheek and strokes the side of her face. 'But I'm glad I found one,' Tanya decides. Pulling the woman closer, moving her mouth over the brunette's lips, she finds her towel falling aside as they lock together in a sudden and passionate embrace.

'You taste of whisky,' the brunette murmurs.

Tanya tests her most seductive smile and says, 'Not everywhere.'

Leonard and Lisa take in the grandeur of the modest pool while holding hands. The temptation to dash to the changing rooms is strong – they are the only couple dressed amongst a dozen or more who are either naked or wearing skimpy towels – but they allow themselves a moment to investigate their surroundings.

Lisa still trembles from her passionate embrace with Kate and the prospect of spending some time in the club with the woman has fuelled a lovely liquid heat deep inside her sex.

After watching his wife and the pretty receptionist enjoy such an obvious kiss, Leonard is struggling to walk without displaying his arousal. He's aware that no one in the swing club will mind if he's sporting an erection but the habits that restrict him outside the club are difficult to shake.

'Swimming or sauna?' Lisa asks.

'Do you want it steamy or wet?'

She smiles at him. And then her attention is caught by the sight of the two women at the side of the pool. Tanya is easy to recognise from the reception area, although most of her face is hidden by the brunette kissing her. Tanya's towel is pooled on the floor beneath her and the new woman she has encountered is eagerly squeezing her large breasts. 'I thought the rules said sex wasn't allowed in the pool?' Lisa frowns.

Leonard shrugs. 'It mentioned something about the filtration system,' he mumbles. 'Maybe it's only men who can't have sex in the pool?' He says no more, not wanting to spoil the atmosphere by painting a detailed word picture of a filtration system clogged with wads of semen.

Tanya's gasp echoes around the hollow acoustics. She arches her back and pushes up her pelvis. As though she is taking this as an invitation, the brunette moves her kisses from Tanya's mouth down to the split between her legs. Her lips glide easily over the woman's bare flesh and then she hesitates above Tanya's sex.

Wordless, enjoying the show and not wanting to spoil the moment, Lisa and Leonard watch. Others around the pool are focusing on the two women. Tony is trying to look casual as he rests against the soft-drinks bar, while another man struggles to conceal his mounting excitement beneath his towel. There are a couple who continue to swim lengths of the pool and remain oblivious to Tanya and her new friend but, aside from them, it does seem as though everyone else in the club is watching.

'Christ! Yes!' Tanya shrieks.

Lisa swallows. 'Lucky bitch,' she murmurs.

Leonard grips her hand tighter.

Tanya lies back, her towel protecting her from the tiled floor surrounding the pool.

'And, besides,' Leonard continues, clearing his throat and trying to resume the conversation from where they'd left off, 'technically, they're not in the pool. They're on the edge.'

Lisa says nothing and, in that silence, Leonard understands she is picturing herself in a similar liaison with Kate. Holding her hand, he can feel the tremors of anticipation bristling through his wife and he relishes her mounting excitement. She is imagining herself as Tanya, with Kate taking the part of the swimmer.

'I thought she came here to suck cock?' Leonard muses.

Lisa shrugs. 'She must have changed her mind. I told her this place is what you make it.'

She continues to watch the two women for a moment longer before slipping her hand from her husband's and then stepping away from him. Blinking his acceptance of this philosophy, Leonard follows Lisa through to the changing rooms.

As the changing-room doors slam closed, Sharon, the brunette swimmer, introduces Tony and Tanya to her partner, Sean. The two men shake hands and compliment each other on their wives.

'They were putting on a good show,' Sean comments.

Tanya glances at the towel he wears around his waist. The front juts noticeably forwards. 'I can see *you* were enjoying it,' she says and smiles.

Uninvited, but confident the action won't be seen as intrusive, she reaches out and circles her hand around his towel-cloaked length. The flesh beneath is hard and thick and she can't suppress the quiver of excitement that touching Sean encourages.

Tony rubs the thrust of his own erection and says, 'I think we were all enjoying it.'

They fall into an easy alliance, Tanya and Sharon comfortably touching each other and Tony and Sean casually discussing the club and how it compares to others they have visited. Throughout the brief chatter of small talk, Tanya's hand remains wrapped around Sean's length and Sharon's fingers continue to play with Tanya's ample breasts.

'Have you seen the playrooms yet?' Sean asks.

Tanya asks quickly, 'Is that an invitation?'

He raises an eyebrow, glances briefly at Tony, and then says, 'Considering the way you're holding me, I didn't think I needed to make a formal invitation.'

Together, the four walk past the sign for the sauna and climb the stairs to the playrooms.

Lisa loses her towel as soon as she steps into the sauna. There is sufficient steam in the small room so that her modesty remains complete but she stills feels a thrill of daring for displaying herself so boldly. The sounds of heavy respiration, thickened by the room's steamy atmosphere, are all around her and she is grateful to know that Leonard is not far behind her.

'Have my seat,' someone gasps. 'It's too damned hot in here for me.'

Lisa thanks the person and squeezes herself on to a bench. Sweaty naked flesh presses against her. Judging by the smoothness of the thigh on her right, and the coarse hairs covering the one on her left, she guesses she is sitting between a man and a woman.

'Are you here on your own?' The question comes from the man on her left. As he speaks, he places his hand lazily on her thigh. The contact is electric enough to make her shiver. She can't see him properly, as the mist is incredibly dense, and it is only when he leans closer that she finds herself smiling at the glowing face of a man ten years her junior.

'I'm here with my husband,' Lisa confesses. She waves a hand into the centre of the sauna and adds, 'I think he's sitting over there, somewhere.'

'He's safe with me,' a woman's voice calls from the other side of the room. Salaciously, she adds, 'Or at least, he's safe for the moment.'

Good-natured chuckles come from the other unseen corners of the room.

Swallowing down her apprehension, throwing herself into the humid spirit of the sauna, Lisa allows the man next to her to trace his fingers higher. Lazily, almost as an afterthought, she places her hand in his lap where her fingers find a thick erection. A crinkle of coarse hairs coats the base of the shaft and she allows her fingertips to explore the sensation of fondling his cock and then his balls.

All the time, she wonders what Leonard might be doing. The woman he's with sounded as youthful as the man to her left. Because Leonard hasn't said anything in response, Lisa wonders if his mouth is otherwise occupied. She pictures him kissing the unseen woman, or suckling against a breast, or kneeling between her open legs and sliding his tongue against her sex lips. Each mental picture is so detailed she can see it in a blaze of vivid colour. And, as her excitement mounts, she grips the man beside her more tightly and begins to slide her curled fist up and down his shaft.

As daring as her, he slips his fingers to the top of her leg and touches the sensitive flesh of her pussy lips.

Lisa draws a startled breath.

'Too much? Too soon?' he asks. Despite the fact he is a stranger, despite the fact that they don't truly know each other, his voice is etched with genuine concern. 'Did I take things too quickly then?' he asks, retrieving his hand.

She shakes her head, and then realises he probably can't see the gesture. Using her right hand to find his, grabbing his wrist and guiding his touch back to her sex lips, she tightens her grip around his shaft. Stroking him slowly up and down, she whispers, 'No. It wasn't too much or too soon. I just hadn't realised it was so hot in here.'

Thrilled by her own daring, she wonders how the man would respond if she were to put her mouth around his erection. The idea sends an absolute shockwave of responses bristling through her.

*　*　*

The erection fills Tanya's mouth, but still she pushes her face forwards and tries to take more. Someone is beneath her, stroking a wet tongue against the sopping lips of her sex, and teasing her to the point of distraction. Her body is alive with so many exciting sensations she feels dizzy with the prospect of orgasm. Staring up at the man above her, wishing he would stop watching his wife and notice how much effort she is putting into sucking the climax from him, Tanya moans to release her frustration and arousal. The room is not what she had been expecting. Lit by a dark-blue bulb, the unfamiliar lighting is disconcerting and throws cold shadows over everyone and everything. Since they entered with Sean and Sharon, other couples have been and gone. Tanya thinks she briefly recognised the couple from reception, although, because she was trying to get two men to come in her mouth at the time, she can't recall if it was really them. A couple to her left are sighing in unison. Words of encouragement, approval and arousal are being murmured like the dialogue from a 70s porn movie.

'You like that, don't you, baby?'
'Take it all the way.'
'You know you want it there.'
'That's it. Squeeze it good and tight.'

Detecting a change in the thickness of the cock in her mouth, Tanya believes she is on the verge of sucking the climax from the man in front of her. Spurred on by the hope of making him come, she works her mouth more quickly up and down his length. A familiar hand grabs her backside. Even with all the distractions, she knows there is only one man in the world who clutches her Daffy Duck with such firm affection. Letting the cock slide from her mouth, she turns to her husband and kisses him hard and passionately. Her mouth is wet from the extra saliva she needed to slide her lips along the sheathed length. And she can feel Tony's arousal increase because he knows she is kissing him with a mouth that has just been wrapped around another man's cock.

In that instant, she is almost pushed beyond the brink of orgasm.

When her lips move away from Tony's, he says, 'Sean and Sharon said to say thank you and goodnight.'

'You've been back to the changing rooms.'

He laughs. 'You can taste the JD on my mouth?'

She grins and turns back to the erection she had been sucking. Her husband takes the initiative and, with her backside presented to him, he pushes the end of his erection against her anus. Tanya grunts, urging her backside back to meet him, and then Tony is slipping into her tight constraints.

For Tanya, the night looks like it is going to be a complete success. She is only sucking on her fourth cock of the evening but, with Tony's erection inside her, and the unknown woman tonguing her pussy, she feels sure the orgasm is going to come quick and strong and provide her with the satisfying memories that she always longs for when attending a swingers' club.

In the pool, Lisa watches Leonard and Sharon kissing. She is chatting amicably with Richard and Rebecca, a couple who come from close to the village in North Wales where she and Leonard live, and Lisa is enjoying the relaxed intimacy. No one is wearing clothes in the pool. Her husband is treating Sharon to a skilful display of his caresses, and Lisa can see that both Richard and Rebecca are sexually interested in her.

'You're bi?' Rebecca asks.

Lisa laughs. 'I'm beginning to think so.'

She remembers sucking on the unseen man's erection in the sauna room. The mental picture is intense and makes her shiver. She hopes the response is hidden by the lapping water that jiggles against her bare breasts.

'And do you swing?' Richard asks.

Lisa nods in the direction of Leonard, who has moved his mouth from Sharon's face and is now kissing her breasts. Her face is contorted into a grimace of ecstasy. 'That's my husband,' Lisa says and smiles. 'He said I wouldn't be allowed to swing with anyone unless he was getting some action too.'

Rebecca giggles.

Richard swims a little closer. His hand moves to Lisa's waist and he leans down to kiss her before continuing with the conversation. His touch is light, sensuous and not intrusive. When Rebecca swims to Lisa's other side, and also places her hand on Lisa's waist, she feels warmed by being a part of the couple's intimacy.

It crosses her mind that she had hoped to encounter Kate, the receptionist, while she was inside the club. The promise of that first kiss has fired her with an arousal that she hasn't yet been able to sate. But, although she feels disappointed that Kate wasn't able to find time to visit the club, Lisa is content to keep company with attentive swingers like Richard and Rebecca.

Moving her mouth from Richard, she turns to Rebecca and kisses her. The exchange is intense and passionate. They embrace, struggling to hold each other and keep their footing in the comparatively shallow end of the pool. When one of them loses their balance, and they both fall under the water, they splutter through water together, laughing and bonding into each other's company. During the cacophony of noise that accompanies their splashing, neither of them hears the receptionist calling Lisa's name.

'Did you have a good night, sweetheart?' Tony asks.

Tanya presses herself into his embrace and nods. 'The best,' she assures him. Despite her smile, she adds, 'But I do feel a bit sorry for that Welsh couple.'

'Leonard and Lisa?'

'Was that their names? I didn't get a chance to talk to them after we met in reception. I'd fancied sucking him off.'

'Why do you feel sorry for them?' Tony asks. 'This isn't one of those Welsh jokes, is it? You're not going to say the club should have a playroom with sheep in it, are you?'

Tanya splutters laughter, tells Tony he is evil and then shakes her head. 'No,' she says, still grinning. 'I just didn't think they got that much out of being there. I didn't see them get off with anyone.'

Tony shrugs and pulls Tanya more tightly into his embrace. His hand drops to her backside and he knows he is holding her directly above her tattoo of Daffy Duck. 'I guess they know the score,' he concedes, no longer caring about the pleasure (or lack of it) that Leonard and Lisa might have enjoyed. 'Didn't she say in reception, it's what you make it?'

Tanya considers this, nods and presses herself into the comfort of her husband's embrace. Dismissing Leonard and Lisa from her thoughts, save for the private promise to look out for them at future clubs and ensure they have a good time if their paths cross again, she looks forward to the night that still lies ahead for her with Tony.

At the reception desk, the young woman who has taken over from Kate stops Leonard and Lisa and asks them for their locker keys. For some reason that Leonard can't fathom, the green that had been so welcoming when they entered now looks cold and seems to encourage them to go. Leonard hands them over, apologising for the oversight.

'Was everything to your satisfaction?'

'Splendid,' Lisa says and grins. 'Although I'm sorry your colleague Kate didn't get a chance to catch up with us in there.'

The receptionist's eyes widen. 'Are you the Welsh lady, Lisa?'

Puzzled, Lisa nods.

The receptionist hands over one of the club's business cards. On the back, Kate has written a telephone number with the message, 'Call me so I can plan to be free the next time you visit.'

Leonard reads the card over his wife's shoulder and then smiles a thank you at the receptionist before leading his wife out of the club.

'What do you make of that?' he asks, as they walk back to their car. 'Is that legitimate? Or just a clever sales tactic?'

Lisa is still studying the business card, wondering if Kate is genuinely interested in seeing her, or if the handwritten number is simply a ploy to encourage repeat custom. She cautions herself for the cynicism, sure it is not warranted, and then slips the business card into the inside pocket of her jacket. 'I don't know,' she muses quietly. Leonard's arm is around her shoulder and she is basking in the warm afterglow that always touches her after such a pleasurable evening. 'I guess it's what you make it.'

WHEN DO YOU SWING?

Considering the way most anecdotes about swinging begin, it's safe to say most first-time occasions take place on a weekend, after the pubs have shut, and when the majority of those involved have imbibed sufficient alcohol to cast aside their inhibitions.

Obviously, swinging can take place at any hour of the day whenever three or more consenting adults have a mind to explore their fantasies. Weekends are more popular with those who are working from Monday to Friday, and holidays do seem a particularly popular time for couples to take things a little further than they have dared during the rest of the year. Again, using the anecdotal evidence that has been gathered in the compilation of this book, it seems many couples enjoy their first swinging experience while holidaying with friends. Reasons for this phenomenon are cited as 'the relaxed atmosphere of a holiday', 'the change of environment' and 'the absence of life's usual pressures'.

Parents who swing, and wish to keep their activities away from perceptive and potentially indiscreet children, are reliant on the services of baby-sitters or understanding relatives. Carefully negotiating their lifestyle around the timetables of others is repeatedly listed as one of the most frustrating aspects of contemporary swinging.

As with every other area of life away from recreational sex, everything from menstrual cycles, unexpected illnesses and demanding work schedules can have an impact on when swingers are able to swing and whether or not they feel the urge to participate.

Swinging clubs report their busiest times between eight o'clock in the evening and one o'clock in the morning. Those who regularly host private parties argue that activities grow more intense after one o'clock. Dogging is more popular in the warmer months, between late spring and early autumn, but even then it usually reaches a peak of activity after dark. Classified adverts enjoy a perennial popularity. Chat rooms for swingers tend to be busier towards the end of the working week as couples and singles arrange to meet over the weekend. Those same rooms are virtually deserted through Saturday and Sunday evening as the swingers enjoy their swinging. But, because of its popularity, 24 hours a day, seven days a week and throughout 365 days of the year, someone, somewhere is certain to be swinging.

Ken

'. . . married women are much better at riding a bloke when they're on top.'

'I wish my current girlfriend was into swinging,' Ken sighs. He delivers this unsolicited sentiment as he sends a text message to his girlfriend telling her he will be spending another Monday evening with friends from the rugby club. The text message is an untruth.

Ken is rapidly approaching his thirties, lives and works in London, and is intimately acquainted with several couples who swing. He spends Wednesday and Friday evenings with his girlfriend while Tuesdays and Thursdays are either at the gym or the rugby field. The weekends are for nightclubs. Monday evenings are invariably taken up with invitations from married friends who invite him to join them in their bedrooms.

'I play with four or five couples at the moment,' Ken explains as he prepares for an evening out. 'The names and faces have changed over the three years since I started swinging, but it's always been roughly around that number.'

In most respects, this is a typical Monday evening for Ken. He will be dining with Gary and Valerie at a North London restaurant and goes through his usual preparations after work. These involve a long soak in the bath, trimming his fingernails and toenails, removing the light scrub of body hair from his chest, stomach and genitals before selecting something smart/casual from his wardrobe. He styles his hair, shaves, scrubs his already immaculate nails, and then tweases away any unsightly hairs from his eyebrows, nostrils and ears. It's a regular Monday-night regime, as disciplined as the practice at his Tuesday rugby training or the sessions he endures each Thursday at the gym.

The final part of Ken's ritual preparation is the liberal application of Hugo Boss.

'Grooming is essential,' he confides. 'Other men's wives expect that.'

On the journey to meet Gary and Valerie, he explains how his first evening with the couple developed.

'First times are usually anxious affairs, but in a good way. I'd met Gary and Valerie through the internet. They suggested we meet up for a drink, and see how things went from there. It's a common arrangement. Valerie is attractive, for an older woman. And I do like older women. While Gary was at the bar getting drinks, I sat beside her and placed my hand on her thigh.'

He laughs and adds, 'It's an unwritten rule of swinging that women wear stockings the first time they meet another person or another couple. Never tights. Never bare legs. Always stockings – nearly always black – and always with a suspender belt.'

Shaking his head to dismiss that detail he says, 'I put my hand on the wife's thigh and that tells me if the couple are really up for it. If the wife doesn't respond, I know she's still got some reservations. If she opens her legs a little, encouraging me to go higher, I know it's game on. The first night I met Gary and Valerie, she opened her legs wide apart.'

He goes on to admit that his first couple of nights with Gary and Valerie did not result in full intimacy. That evening involved Ken and Valerie kissing and touching while Gary watched and masturbated. Their second evening only saw them undressing each other with Gary again remaining in the corner of the room.

'Gary and Valerie like to play it slow,' he explains. 'But we all get on together and I don't mind whether I play slow or fast. I particularly like seeing this couple because we all respect each other's boundaries. I've seen them about ten times now and they always want to take things a little bit further. They're a lot of fun to be with and I feel honoured that they've shared this part of their lives with me.'

The last thing he says before leaving for his meal with the couple is an echo of the melancholy refrain he mentioned before: 'I really wish my current girlfriend was into swinging. We could really have some fun if she was into swinging.'

Gary and Valerie are waiting for Ken at the restaurant. They enjoy a quiet meal together, catching up with events in each other's lives before discussing the way they would like this evening to progress. Because Valerie and Ken are sitting close together, they are able to touch between courses and whenever they think their actions will go unnoticed by the restaurant's staff and clientele.

Under the table, his fingers move up her thigh and beneath her skirt. He touches the warm, moist crotch of her panties. Valerie touches the bulge at the front of Ken's pants. Gary watches the half-concealed fumbling with an indulgent smile.

The atmosphere between the three is one of playful expectation. Valerie has fixed ideas about what she wants to happen this evening and she coyly alludes to some of the things she would like to do with Ken. Teasing her, Ken feigns ignorance and says she will have to whisper her needs if she wants him to understand. Valerie blushes, cups her hand over his ear, and tells Ken that she wants him to take 'explicit' photographs of her and Gary. She also wants Gary to be 'surprised' each time he returns to the room and discovers they have become 'intimate' without him being there. Ken pretends he doesn't understand what she means by 'explicit' and 'intimate' and presses her to state her needs in vulgar terms. When Valerie eventually relents, he then appears comically shocked by her coarse language. Although Valerie is twenty years Ken's senior, they joke together as though they are peers on a first date.

Their time at the restaurant is an extension of the foreplay the trio always enjoy when they meet up and Ken admits it is a similar relationship to that which he shares with some of his other married friends.

Valerie and Ken touch and kiss and surreptitiously tease. Gary exchanges loving glances with his wife. He watches her with obvious affection and excitement. As the group are finishing their coffees at the end of the meal, Gary politely asks Ken if he wants to come back home with them. It's a formality they've carried with them since their first meeting and is a coded way of asking if they all want to proceed with the planned evening, or if anyone wants to decline from going any further. Ken readily agrees. Valerie also gives her approval.

'I adore married women,' Ken admits. 'Especially those who swing. They hold themselves with so much confidence. They know what they want. And married women are much better at riding a bloke when they're on top.'

Gary drives them home from the restaurant. Valerie and Ken sit in the back of the car and continue touching and teasing each other. Their mouths are constantly locked in a kiss and Ken has managed to slip a hand inside her blouse to touch the bare flesh of her breast.

The play stops as soon as they reach Gary and Valerie's home in Hadley Wood. Cautious of the neighbours seeing anything, very concerned about their reputation, Gary and Valerie have told Ken that nothing untoward must be seen on the walk from the car (parked on the driveway) to the front door. Valerie straightens her clothes, as she and Ken climb out of the car using separate doors, and they don't resume any contact until they are inside the house and the door is closed and locked behind them. It is another of the rituals with which they are all now familiar.

'Different couples like to do things in different ways,' Ken explains. 'I used to see this one pair who were the exact opposite of Gary and Valerie. They would have been happy for us to do it on the front lawn during broad daylight in front of a street party. I've been with other couples who have just one fixed scenario in their minds and they keep coming back to it until it's so boring it's repetitive. Sometimes the husband wants to watch his wife get fucked by another guy, and then they can't wait to get rid of me once I've done my part. There are also others, where the wife will really rip on her husband while we're fucking, telling him he's incompetent or impotent and useless. And that can be kind of off-putting.

'That's one of the reasons I like Gary and Valerie. They plan everything out in advance and they're always thoughtful enough to include me in the planning. If my girlfriend ever came round to the idea of swinging, I'd like to think we could be like Gary and Valerie.'

Inside the house, Gary goes to find his camera equipment, and organise drinks for the three of them. Valerie and Ken retire to a downstairs room and make themselves comfortable on the settee.

'Our first sessions were fairly tame,' Ken admits. 'Valerie and I kissed and touched a lot but didn't take it much further. Since then, we've been making up for lost time and it's almost customary for us to spend as much time as we can getting physical. Usually, when Gary's joined us in the lounge, I'm sat on the settee and Valerie has her mouth around my cock.'

This evening is no exception and, when Gary returns, Valerie smiles at her husband while she is sucking another man's erection. Although he is distracted by events, even Ken can see the pair are both stimulated by this silent exchange.

The photographs they are taking are intended for an internet dating site and Ken gets the couple to pose individually, together, and then while they're engaged in intercourse. Valerie and Gary wear dark glasses to preserve some anonymity and the digital camera means they have no need to get the photographs developed by a third party. Valerie takes advantage of the opportunity to try on a variety of lingerie and repeatedly solicits Ken's opinion as to which looks best.

After Ken has taken sufficient photographs to fill the camera, Valerie sends Gary to their computer room, telling him to upload the images to their PC while she and Ken share a drink.

'Usually we'll have sex three or four times on an evening,' Ken explains. 'That means I'll be with them for three or four hours and I'll come three or four times. I'm not trying to make myself out as a super stud. But I am fit and healthy. And I do find the situation of being involved with a couple to be very arousing.'

When Gary returns, with the camera ready for use again, he finds his wife is on the floor with Ken. Valerie is wearing stockings and a bra and she is riding Ken vigorously. Her feet are placed firmly on the carpet and she squats over him while rolling her pelvis. Both are clearly enjoying the intimacy and Valerie seems delighted that she has again been 'caught' by her husband.

Putting the photography aside for the moment, Gary joins the pair and has Valerie suck his erection while she continues to ride Ken.

The drinks they enjoy are invariably soft ones. Neither Gary nor Valerie is a big drinker and Ken doesn't like to overindulge when he is with a couple. The sobriety does not extend to their moods though and, as the passion escalates, Valerie gets a fit of the giggles and Gary and Ken join in her mirth.

Gary ejaculates in his wife's mouth. Valerie and Ken achieve their orgasms at roughly the same time. As the three of them gather their strength for another bout of intimacy, Gary takes a few more photographs of Valerie.

The conversation that has been flowing all night continues. Gary and Valerie ask Ken about the other couples he visits and Ken enquires about their encounters with other singles and couples. Valerie seems keen to find out what Ken's other friends demand of him, and he is eager to know if there is anything they have tried that he has yet to enjoy. Because the topic of conversation remains fixed on swinging, swapping and general sexual preferences, all three enjoy a high mood of arousal. Gary retires from the room twice more to upload fresh photos of his wife, and Ken and Valerie manage to 'surprise' him each time he returns.

It is after midnight before Ken is taking a taxi ride home and assuring his girlfriend, via text message, that he has had a good evening with his friends from the rugby club.

After the high spirits he has enjoyed with Gary and Valerie, he seems comparatively subdued. 'I do wish my current girlfriend was into swinging,' he admits. 'I know the husbands seem to get a lot from seeing their wives with another man. And I think I can understand how they get that pleasure. From what the wives I've met tell me, the experience is great for them. And I believe my girlfriend would really enjoy it.

'However, every time I've raised the subject, she's dismissed the whole lifestyle as perverted and wrong. So it's unlikely it's going to happen for us.' He laughs with sour amusement and adds, 'It feels odd to be the single man going to see a couple, and know that I'm the only one there who is technically cheating on someone.'

This concern about his lack of fidelity seems real and genuine. But it doesn't stop Ken from sending Gary and Valerie a text message to thank them for the fun evening and to enquire if they will be seeing each other next Monday.

Sam & Sandra
'. . . adventurous couple seeks similar . . .'

'It's a surprise.' The solemnity of Sam's words are spoilt by the mischievous twinkle in his eyes. Sandra wants to ask him more but, because they are at a conventional party, attended by family and friends, she knows this is not the right time or place to press him for details. The village pub is busy; a buffet has been laid along one side of the bar and a banner hangs over the bar proclaiming 'HAPPY 40TH'. Sam and Sandra's conversation is loud enough to carry over the strumming of the band as they warm up ready to play.

Acting the role of the petulant birthday girl, frowning childishly and getting ready to throw a fake tantrum, Sandra says, 'It's my birthday *today* and I want my surprise *now*.'

A nearby relative chuckles. Most likely it's Aunt Caroline. After two gins, she chuckles at anything. Sandra's best friend, Linda, murmurs something about Sandra regressing to a second childhood now she's reached forty. While the comment is harsh, Sandra knows it has been said in fun.

'You can't have your present now,' Sam tells Sandra. He uses the same tone of voice that is usually reserved for telling their children they are not allowed a particular game for the PlayStation. 'Your surprise is organised for *next* weekend.'

'That is so unfair!' Sandra exclaims.

Sam raises an eyebrow and glances towards their children. They are sitting patiently with their grandparents and, for once, not causing the mayhem that has turned his hair prematurely grey at the temples. 'Do you think this sort of behaviour is setting a good example to our offspring?'

'I learnt this behaviour from them,' Sandra retorts.

The remark breaks the tension that has been building. As though prompted to deliver a rejoinder, the three children wail in protest at the slur Sandra has cast in their direction. Those who have witnessed the small scene laugh loudly and the mirth is then replaced by the sounds of chatter, drinking and general conversation. The band take this moment to start their set and the pub quietens beneath the lull of Sandra's favourite rock ballad: Aerosmith's 'Don't want to Miss a Thing'. Sam and Sandra embrace and move towards the dance floor. As they smooch slowly together, she presses her lips to his ear and asks, 'Is it the same sort of surprise as last year?'

'That would be telling,' he demurs. 'But the answer to that one is yes.'

She shivers against him. And they both know the tremor was inspired by a thrill of sexual excitement.

'We've been married for fifteen years this December,' Sam explains. He is 45, dresses like an executive in a suit, collar and tie, and the silver hair at his temples makes him look distinguished.

Sandra says, 'We started talking about swinging after five years of marriage.' Recently turned forty, Sandra wears jeans and a large England sweatshirt, as though she is on her way to collect the children from school. Her blonde hair has been hurriedly pulled into a grip and, although dishevelled, manages to look casually elegant. 'But,' she continues, 'it took another five years before we grew a big enough pair to do something about it.'

Sam continues from Sandra's interjection. 'At first we tried classified ads.'

'We were "adventurous couple seeks similar",' Sandra declares proudly.

'And we met some interesting people,' Sam concludes.

'Then we tried a couple of clubs and parties,' Sandra continues. 'And they were a giggle too.'

'But the biggest hurdle for us,' Sam explains, 'is time management.'

'What he means,' Sandra elaborates, 'is that we always struggle to find time for swinging when we're not working, meeting up with family or non-swinging friends, or doing something with the kids.'

They explain that the idea of swinging came through discussions of how they could keep the spark of arousal within their sex life. After trying every different sexual position their bodies could assume, and following the vanilla guidelines suggested by the mainstream agony aunts, which included lingerie, sexual surprises and massage, Sam suggested they should try wife-swapping. Sandra was intrigued by the idea – she hadn't dared suggest that particular avenue herself – and from that day onwards a variety of potential scenarios began to dominate their sexual fantasies.

Five years later, their swinging lifestyle was still a fantasy and Sandra boldly suggested they should make it a reality. Following an ordeal of conversations where they each assured the other that sleeping with different partners would not undermine their mutual love or respect, they placed their first advert declaring 'adventurous couple seeks similar'.

'We had a pretty good idea of what we wanted from swinging,' Sam confides.

Sandra corrects him. 'After five years of talking about it in the bedroom, we knew *exactly* what we wanted from swinging. The recurring theme to our fantasies was that I wanted to be the centre of attention for at least two men and Sam wanted to watch.'

'But, still,' Sam continues, 'we kept struggling to organise the swinging around more important commitments. There's never a choice between making a date with a new couple or tending to the needs of the family. Family always comes first. The only exception is Sandra's birthday. Every year, for the past five years, I have always scheduled time so she has the opportunity for a special birthday treat.'

Grinning broadly, Sandra says, 'He excelled himself for my fortieth.'

A week after her fortieth birthday party, with Sandra waving goodbye to the children as Sam drives their Volvo slowly out of the cul-de-sac, she asks, 'So what's the surprise?'

'You're less than two hours away from finding out,' Sam reminds her. 'Do you really want me to spoil things for you now?'

She considers her answer for a moment before saying, 'Yes.'

'Well, I won't.'

'Does it involve sex?'

'I told you to put stockings on, didn't I?'

'You're always telling me to put stockings on. You're a sick and twisted pervert.' This refers to a long-running joke between the couple: Sam continually asks his wife to wear stockings because he maintains they emphasise her beautiful legs and perpetually remind her she is desirable; Sandra insists he likes her to wear them because he's a lech.

'So it does involve sex?'

'If everything works out as planned, there's a good chance it will involve sex.'

'Who with?'

Shaking his head, unable to contain his smile, Sam turns on the car's radio and steers the Volvo towards the motorway. The journey takes little more than an hour and Sandra is not surprised when Sam pulls the Volvo into the car park of a familiar motel. It is a discreet location that they have used several times previously when they've been meeting couples and singles.

As soon as they arrive, Sam asks his wife to make herself comfortable in their room while he sorts out 'some business' at the bar. Sensing the seriousness of his tone – and now touched by a thrill of anticipation – Sandra does as he has suggested.

Thirty minutes later, alone in the motel bedroom, Sandra sits apprehensively on the edge of the bed sipping a nasty cup of tea. She is dressed in stockings, a thong and a filmy wrap that clings to her bare breasts. The predominant colour of her lingerie is a delicate baby pink. Set off by her slender body and blonde hair, the pastel colour makes her look younger than her forty years and, she hopes, more desirable.

The delay between leaving Sam in the motel's bar has now grown intolerably long and Sandra is beginning to wonder if his plans have not panned out. Too many of their potential swinging escapades have ended in a frustrating disappointment. As she is aware from her own perspective, family can inadvertently interfere, too often couples simply lose their nerve, and occasionally things just happen so that the swinging doesn't work out. Because this is an adventure Sam has planned for her birthday, Sandra silently prays that she is only suffering a delay from her surprise and not a cancellation.

A knock on the door startles her from her thoughts and she almost spills the cup of insipid motel tea she has been drinking. Not sure what to expect, wishing Sam had given her some indication of what her birthday surprise might be, she rushes to the door, takes a deep breath, and then opens it a tentative quarter of an inch.

'Hello?'

'Sandra?'

'Yes.'

'We've just been with Sam in the bar. He said he'd be along shortly. But he thought we should come up here and introduce ourselves.'

Sandra opens the door another quarter of an inch, still unable to see who is standing in the hall. It's a woman's voice talking to her but she is speaking in the plural, evidently not alone. Cautious – curious but not wanting to do anything with foolish haste – Sandra asks, 'Did Sam give you a message for me?'

'He said we should wish you a happy birthday.'

Sandra opens the door. She finds herself staring at a young blonde who stands in front of two large, grinning black men. Her heart begins to race.

'I don't like to talk about my fantasies of having sex with a black man,' Sandra admits. She blushes and the colour rises quickly in her cheeks. 'I worry that I might come across as being racist. I don't consider myself racist, and I don't think I'm trying to exploit anyone. I just fancy doing it with a black guy because I know it would be different.'

'Well,' Sam says dryly. 'You've made that crystal clear.'

She fixes him with a withering glare and elaborates. 'I'm not suggesting it would feel different. And I'm not stupid enough to believe that it's true about black guys having bigger cocks. I just think it would be different to see my pale body in the embrace of a jet-black man. Different and, therefore, exciting. I think the experience of swinging is fantastic. I love to have sex with other men as well as with my husband. But I think having sex with someone of a different colour would make that difference more appreciable. I think that's why I have always wanted the experience.'

'The swingers we've met have been a fairly WASP bunch,' Sam explains. 'I don't know if it's because swinging is mainly a WASP thing, or if non-whites have their own swinging circles that we've never encountered because we're not non-whites.'

'The few parties and clubs we've been to where there have been black guys, the poor bastards have been swamped,' Sandra interjects. 'And, although I've always hankered for a bit of black, Sam and I have never specifically advertised for a black couple because I've always said it sounds tacky.'

Sam grins, places a hand on his wife's arm and says, 'For her birthday, I posted a tacky advert.'

The blonde girl is called Gillian and she is married to Frank, the taller of the two men she introduces. The other man is Frank's brother, Dean, and he closes the door as Sandra invites them into the room.

'Are you sure this is the right room?' Frank asks, appraising Sandra. 'Your husband said we were here to help you celebrate your fortieth birthday. And you don't look forty to me.'

Sandra laughs. Smiling at Gillian, she says, 'He's divine. I could kiss him already.'

Shrugging easily, Gillian takes off her coat and says, 'You can do more than kiss him. I don't think he'll object.'

The comment turns the air to syrup. Sandra's apprehension vanishes as her mood shifts to raw arousal. Turning to face Frank, she feels small and vulnerable beneath his large towering frame. When he steps nearer, and places an arm around her waist so he can pull her close, she wants to swoon against him.

Frank kisses her with an overt familiarity. His lips crush against hers and his tongue slips easily into her mouth. With another couple – and particularly if Sam was in the room – Sandra knows the introductory period would be stretched out with handshakes, greetings and small-talk questions about the journey, the weather and the latest headlines. Because Sam has yet to join them, and because Frank seems quite happy to dictate the tempo of how this afternoon is going to continue, Sandra allows him to press his body against her as the kiss becomes more urgent.

'I don't know which one of you is more ready for it,' Gillian says, laughing.

'I reckon it's Frank,' Dean breaks in. Glancing at Gillian, he says, 'Frank was horny on the journey down here; he was begging you to blow him while he drove.'

Sandra pulls herself away from the kiss and glances at Gillian. 'And did you?'

Gillian shakes her head.

Smiling hungrily, Sandra teases a finger against the front of Frank's jeans and chases the shape of his erection. 'If you didn't blow him,' she begins coyly, 'perhaps I should do the honours before we properly begin?'

In reply, Gillian fetches a fruit-flavoured condom from her purse and passes it to Sandra.

A quarter of an hour later, when Sam steps into the room and has observed the event has started without him, he takes an order for drinks and goes back to the bar. When he returns, his wife is in the centre of the bed and kneeling on all fours. Dean is in her mouth, while Frank is sliding in and out of her in a doggy-style and Gillian lounges in a nearby chair with her legs spread wide apart as she fingers herself.

The afternoon progresses slowly, Gillian and Sam only watching and masturbating, while Dean, Frank and Sandra fuck in a variety of positions. Her hunger for the two men appears insatiable and she takes them repeatedly between her legs and in her mouth, constantly calling for more.

The contrast between their dark bodies and Sandra's pale flesh is startling. Sam is particularly struck by the image of Dean's short thick erection plunging between Sandra's sex. Watching the dark man's heavy black balls pounding against his wife's parchment-pale buttocks, he has to stop stroking himself for fear of climaxing too soon.

Sandra takes both men in her mouth at the same time and then tries to organise a double penetration from them both. They are three hours into the day and her body is slick with sweat and her hair is plastered to her scalp. The neatly made motel room is in complete disarray as the bed linen looks rumpled and tables and furniture have been shifted to make various positions more accessible for Dean, Frank and Sandra or more visible for Gillian and Sam.

Sandra coaxes Dean to lie on the bed and then she straddles him as though they are going to enjoy a variation on the missionary position. As soon as his sheathed length is inside her sex, she summons Frank and tries to wedge his erection into her anus.

Whether it's because of his weariness, her own inability to guide him straight, or some other factor, she can't manage to squeeze his thickness into the tight hole of her backside. Groaning with frustration, she releases her hold on Frank and writhes against Dean until a final climax is wrung from her body. Even as she is shivering through the final part of the orgasm, and although it's obvious she is exhausted, Sandra immediately turns around and sucks Frank to a final climax for the day.

Still sitting side by side – neither touching the other but both watching exactly the same scene – Gillian and Sam climax in unison.

Later that day, after saying farewell to Gillian, her husband and her brother-in-law, Sandra and Sam order a pizza to their room, a couple more drinks from the bar and curl up in the bed together. They are both exhausted and satisfied.

'Thank you,' Sandra whispers. 'It was a lovely surprise and even better than last year's.'

He laughs and kisses her. 'It's kind of you to say that, but you haven't had *all* the surprise yet.'

Sandra stares at him, puzzled by the remark, her tin of lager and her pizza briefly forgotten. 'What else have you organised? What have you been planning?'

'I haven't organised much more,' Sam confesses, 'but I did ask Gillian if she, Dean and Frank would care to join us tomorrow, so we could all play again.'

'What did they say?' Sandra demands. She is sitting up, vibrant, alert and desperate to hear his answer. 'What did they say?'

Sam shakes his head, his smile glinting mischievously. 'I won't tell you now,' he decides. 'It will spoil the surprise.'

Walter & Wendy
'I'm being ravaged by some sort of wild animal!'

A huge full moon dominates the inky sky. Despite its silver glow, it throws little light on the countryside below and only shapes the shadows and silhouettes. Twin beams from an Audi cut through the night and glide smoothly around tight bends and along narrow curves. The air outside the car is cool enough to leave a sheen of mist on the windscreen. And, as they spot the sign indicating a lay-by 100 yards ahead, George and Glenda exchange a nervous glance.

'Do you still want to?'

Glenda is aghast. 'We can't just drive past.'

'I'm just saying, if you want to back out, now would be the ideal time.'

She considers nodding, allowing George to hit the accelerator and drive past the woman waiting at the lay-by they are approaching. The image is easy to conjure up – it comes with such clarity she can picture the disappointed frown on Wendy's face – then Glenda quickly shakes her head and refuses that option. 'I don't want to back out. Do you?'

'No. I was just giving you the option.'

Glenda points. 'Oh! Look over there.' Her voice has suddenly turned theatrical, as though she is reciting pre-scribed lines from a text. 'There's a woman in the lay-by trying to flag us down. It looks like she's got a flat tyre.'

Checking his rear-view mirror, then indicating as he eases his foot on the brake, George mumbles, 'Now there's a fucking surprise.'

Glenda fixes him with a glare and he mumbles an apology.

The Audi pulls in behind the parked Toyota and, in the glow of the headlights, they can see the woman waiting there is in her late forties and dressed as though she was interrupted on her way to a party.

'We have a very specific fantasy that we like to play out,' Walter explains. 'Which is why our swinging is limited to three nights of the month. We meet couples mainly through classified adverts in magazines and newspapers, although Wendy is taking computer courses now because a couple of people we've met say the internet is a good place to meet up and make contacts.'

At the age of 52, Walter's thick-set beard and unruly brown hair make him look a lot older. While it may sound unkind, the word 'grizzled' is the first one that leaps to mind when trying to describe him. He dresses in a plaid work shirt and tired denims, and the clothes make his appearance large, bulky and formidable. With the sleeves of his shirt rolled up, he exposes brawny forearms that are thick with dark curly hair. His shirt is open at the collar and reveals similar curls up to his throat.

By contrast to Walter's rural appearance, Wendy dresses as though she is trying to compensate for her husband's lack of elegance. Her dress fits snugly. The hem exposes the knees of her stocking-clad legs and has a neckline that plunges deep to reveal an inviting cleavage. She wears a flimsy stole over her bare shoulders. Aside from the plain band on her wedding finger, her only jewellery is a necklace weighted by a pendant that looks like a silver bullet.

'Our fantasy begins on the night of a full moon. Wendy is alone and stuck in a remote lay-by. She flags down a couple, thanks them for stopping, and then asks them for their help.'

'Thank goodness you stopped,' Wendy exclaims. 'I really do need your help.'

'It looks like you've had a blow-out,' Glenda says, climbing out of the car.

It doesn't really look like Wendy has had a blow-out. The Toyota stands on four plump tyres and has no discernible problems other than a little rust over the rear arches. But, because Walter and Wendy have provided the couple with a suggested script for the fantasy, she provides the lines that they gave her. It is October but the night isn't as cold as she had expected. A thin gauze of mist that weights the air makes Glenda pull her fleece more tightly around her shoulders.

'Do you want us to get some help?'

'Didn't we pass a castle back down the road a few miles?' George breaks in. 'Maybe they have a telephone I might use.'

Glenda glares at him, aware that he is quoting from the *Rocky Horror Picture Show* and annoyed that he is not taking the couple's fantasy seriously. 'No, we didn't pass a fucking castle back down the road,' she snaps.

'And I'd rather you didn't leave me here alone,' Wendy adds earnestly. She places a hand on George's forearm, clutching him tight and moving close. Her gaze is widened by a haunted expression. 'I'm not sure it's safe out here,' she whispers. 'There's something lurking nearby.'

'What makes you think it's not safe?'

'Something attacked me before you arrived.' Wendy's haunted expression turns briefly wild as she glances around the blackness that surrounds them. 'If we can go in the back seat of your car, I'll show you the marks it made on me.'

'It?' Glenda asks. 'You make it sound like you were attacked by some sort of creature or wild animal.'

Wendy is already leading George to the Audi. Calling over her shoulder, she tells Glenda, 'It *was* a wild animal. It was very, very wild indeed.'

'We meet up first and get to know the couple over a drink or two at a local pub,' Walter explains. 'When you've met a person in the flesh, so to speak, you get a good idea of whether or not they're ready to play. And it gives them a chance to decide whether our fantasy scenario is the sort of thing that they want to try, or whether it's not something that turns them on.'

'Not every couple wants to play along with our fantasy,' Wendy admits. 'But that's OK because I'm sure we wouldn't want to try some of the fantasies that other people have.'

'Over a couple of pints and a half-hour chat, we've usually got an idea whether or not a couple want to try our game. That's when we tell them what we fancy and they either agree to give it a try, or tell us that it's not for them.'

Wendy nods and turns around to proudly display her left shoulder. She slips the shawl away as she moves. 'I've had this done to make our fantasy that little bit more real for us.'

Walter smiles proudly, as she shows off the tattoo. Drawn in red and purple inks, the design is fashioned to make it look as though her shoulder blade has been torn open by four deep gouges from a heavily clawed hand. The artist has done an impressive job, colouring the picture so it looks bloody and open, suggesting bruised muscle tissue in the centre of the design beneath ravaged strips of skin, and even shading the areas around the tattoo to give depth to the image of lacerations.

George stares at the claw mark on Wendy's left shoulder. His fingers trace lightly over the smooth flesh that has been decorated to look like an injury. Wendy's skin is cool beneath his caress but he can feel that she is ready to respond to him. The prospect stirs a slow rush of warmth to his loins. Remembering his script for the evening he tries to sound genuinely shocked as he asks, 'What the hell did this to you?'

'I'm not sure.' Wendy's tone is rich with the breathless theatrics of someone who devotes their free time to amateur dramatics. Beneath her stilted words, she also sounds as though she is trying to contain a mounting arousal. 'Everything happened so fast, and it was too dark for me to see properly.' She turns and places a modest hand over her ample bosom. Because she has unfastened her dress to show off the mark on her shoulder, her breasts are only covered by her arm. She regards George warily and asks, 'Would you check the rest of my body and see if the creature scratched anywhere else?'

Without waiting for his answer, she slips out of her dress and reveals herself naked save for a pair of black stockings. The interior light of the car is flattering and disguises the paunch of her stomach and the sag of her breasts. Leaning close to George, placing her lips so they hover over his, Wendy whispers, 'Examine me thoroughly. Its claws were all over me and I want to make sure that I've not been damaged.'

Manfully, George pushes her back on to the Audi's rear seat. He lowers his face to one breast. Moving forwards he plants his knees between her spread thighs. He hesitates before placing his lips around her stiff nipple and growls, 'This is the best way I know of finding out whether a woman has been damaged.'

And then he lowers his mouth to take one thick nipple between his lips and begins to suck. Wendy moans as he teases her. Eagerly, she pushes her pelvis up to meet his groin. The urgency of her need is infectious and George can feel his erection straining to be released and satisfied. One of Wendy's hands rests on his back, pulling him closer to her. The other is at his groin, rubbing the thickening flesh of his cock.

'I haven't examined you down there yet,' he says quickly. 'I was going to use my tongue for that.'

'This will be a better way of doing the examination,' Wendy assures him. She pulls at his trousers and manages to tear the zip open. Reaching inside the open fly, her cool fingers encircle the warm heat of his hardness.

Through the Audi's open door, Glenda watches her husband suckle against Wendy. The sight is infuriatingly exciting and she crushes her thighs together. Seeing the woman eager for her husband, watching Wendy pull him closer and then fumble to free his cock from his pants, Glenda is struck by the same sting of excitement that always hits her when she and George are with another couple. Her nipples are hard inside her blouse and her sex feels sticky with heat.

The scene is mesmerising enough to make her weak and oblivious to the stealthy figure creeping up behind her. She watches Wendy drag George's erection from his trousers, stroke the foreskin back and then slide a condom over the glans with a speed that is enviably swift. After rolling the sheath down his length with an effortless flick of her wrist, Wendy grabs the base of George's erection and guides him towards the open split of her sex.

Glenda trembles as she watches her husband push inside the woman. She is still shivering when someone grabs her from behind and drags her to the front of the car. Pushed over the bonnet of the Audi – breathless, surprised and now anxious for satisfaction – she gasps but makes no other protest. Her skirt is pulled up to her waist and the crotch of her panties is tugged aside. The lack of foreplay and the vigorous handling is more of an aphrodisiac than she had thought it would be. Also, the silence of the man behind her is another spur to her arousal. Instead of speaking or trying to excite her with flattery, he is merely grunting and panting and determined to have her over the bonnet of the car.

Hurriedly, he ingratiates himself between her legs and pushes her thighs apart. His fingers scratch against her buttocks, heightening her warmth and increasing her excitement. Although she can't see, Glenda knows the split of her sex is open and wet and ready for the man behind her.

The night is cool but not cold – her pussy lips feel as though they are melting in contrast to the air that brushes them – and she knows the excitement of having watched her husband with Wendy has warmed the centre of her sex. Now she wants her excitement satisfied by Walter and his unusual fantasy.

'Who are you?' she croaks. 'And what do you think you're doing to me?'

Rather than reply, Walter simply pushes his hips forwards so the end of his hardness prods the top of her thighs.

Walter is not attractive but Glenda has to admit he is the ideal person to play the role of the marauding werewolf in this fantasy. The arms that hold her to the bonnet of the car are strong and covered with sufficient excess hair to give him a lycanthropic appearance. The bearded face that presses kisses against the back of her neck feels like the muzzle of a wild and unkempt animal. And his erection is trying to force itself between her legs.

The excitement of the moment grows stronger. She doesn't know if Walter is wearing a condom and, at the moment, Glenda is beyond caring. His length feels smooth enough to be sheathed and that's as much precaution as she feels in the mood to take. As he pushes forwards, her sex welcomes him in a warm and fluid rush. The thickness is greater than she expected and the surge of pleasure flowing through her is a lot more forceful than she anticipated.

Walter pushes in and out vigorously, riding her with little thought for the pleasure he might be providing and still staying in character with his animal grunts and groans. She briefly frets that he might hurt her by pressing her so hard against the bonnet or pushing into her with such vicious and brutal thrusts. And then Glenda remembers that she was excited by the fantasy Walter and Wendy had suggested and wants to feel a man who is a little more forceful than her caring husband.

She allows the surge of pleasure to flow freely through her body. Her breasts are warmed by the car's bonnet and she can feel her nipples growing hard enough to possibly scratch the metalwork. Walter is still behind her and he makes each thrust hard enough to shake the Audi.

Eventually, after a rush of pleasure has built inside her body, Glenda remembers that she has to call for help to make the fantasy seem convincing. 'George,' she cries weakly. 'You have to come quick. You have to come quick because something has got me. I'm being ravaged by some sort of wild animal!'

Behind her, as he pushes his erection between her legs, Walter howls like a wolf.

'We'd played the werewolf game a few times before we thought about inviting another couple to join us. It's always been a bit daring because we're on the side of the road, and you never know who might come driving past.'

'We did get spotted once by a car,' Wendy says and grins. 'And that was what caused us to start talking about inviting another couple to play. Walter had me bent over the bonnet of our Toyota – he was taking me really roughly from behind – and I don't think either of us noticed that this car was coming down on us. The next we knew they were driving past, honking their horn and shouting a couple of things out of the window. I think it was encouragement.' She shakes her head and adds, 'It was embarrassing in some ways. We were both naked, which meant they got to see my breasts and my private parts, and Walter's backside. I'd say his private parts too but, at the time, he'd got them hidden inside me.'

'When we got back, we started talking about what we'd have done if they'd stopped and come over,' Walter explains. 'We both said it would have been shameful but Wendy said it would also have been exciting if they'd wanted to join in. We bought a contact magazine the following day and started looking for another couple to join us.'

'Don't go out there,' Wendy exclaims theatrically.

Buried between her thighs, enjoying the sensation of taking her on the back seat of the car, as his wife groans with obvious pleasure outside, George has no intention of getting out of the car. He lowers his mouth back to her breast and continues to ride in and out of Wendy's wetness. When she moans and grabs his back, hungrily pulling him closer and pushing her sex more fully around his length, George struggles to contain the climax that has been building in his loins.

'I'm not going out there yet,' he says heroically. 'I'll leave Glenda to tackle that beast while you deal with this one.' Forcefully, he pushes himself deeper inside her.

Groaning with arousal, Wendy releases her own wolflike howl. The sound is ear-splitting in the confines of the car.

'We work our fantasy to a script,' Walter explains. 'That way, things don't go off in a direction none of us is expecting.'

Wendy nods agreement. 'The whole thing starts when I thank the couple for stopping and ask them if they can help me.'

'And,' Walter breaks in, 'it marks the beginning of the end when the man from the other couple asks me to take Wendy to my harem.'

'Try this one,' George says, helping Wendy from the car. 'She's called Wendy.'

Walter studies George warily. Slowly, he pulls his erection from Glenda's sex. Glenda moans. Her features are strained into a mask of frustration and George can see his wife is close to achieving a sorely needed climax. While he was riding Wendy, he felt sure he had heard Glenda shriek her way through at least one climax and he is pleasantly surprised by her appetite for more. Anxious to be inside her when she achieves her next orgasm, desperate to pleasure his wife and feel the special bond of satisfaction that they always share when they have been swinging with another couple, he coaxes Wendy to go to Walter's side and reaches out to take Glenda in his embrace.

'You can have this one for your harem, Wolfman,' George tells Walter. He pushes Wendy towards the hirsute figure and nods at Glenda. 'I'll have this one for my harem.'

'Do you think you can service this one well?' Walter asks, placing a hand against Glenda's exposed backside. He speaks like someone auditioning for the role of Tarzan. His fingers linger close to her pussy lips.

'Why don't we service them together, before we go our separate ways?' George suggests. He pulls Glenda to the driver's side of the bonnet and encourages Walter to take Wendy over the passenger side.

The two men push into their respective partners and, together, as they pound urgently into their women, all four of them howl in unison. The sound trails easily over the midnight landscape and is then lost in the all-consuming darkness that surrounds them.

'Ordinary swinging has never appealed to us,' Walter confides. 'Without the addition of our fantasy scene, the sex seems to be lacking something. We've taken up suggestions from other couples and tried sharing and swapping without my having a full moon or Wendy having her ravaging fantasy, but it's never quite the same.'

Wendy nods agreement. 'Ours is a fantasy that we can only bring to life during the full moon,' she explains. She grins at her husband with obvious affection and says, 'It's the full moon that brings out the animal in him.'

WHY DO YOU SWING?

The arguments against swinging are an unavoidable part of our cultural conditioning. The immorality of sexual pleasure is reinforced by peer pressure and the doctrine of most mainstream religions. The quest for successful monogamy has been the subtext of every romance novel ever written. Media representations of swingers denigrate participants for their unconventional lifestyles and subversive ethics. The threat of exposure and subsequent condemnation make this deviation from the norm seem like too great a risk for too little reward. Coupled with the worry of disease; fears of failure, rejection and inadequacy, as well as the dark pall of secrecy shrouding recreational sex, it is far easier to understand why people *don't* swing.

But active participants present many strong arguments for their lifestyle. Alan and Jennifer, a swinging Midlands couple, explained they had become involved to accommodate Jennifer's bisexuality in their relationship. Alan says, 'We didn't see why the fact that we were in a relationship now had to mean that she was to close off half her sexuality, and so we were open to the idea of a non-exclusive relationship from the start.'

Swingers throughout the country confirm that female bisexuality is common within the community. Although male bisexuality seldom features at swingers' parties, experiments between women are regular occurrences.

Lisa and Leonard, a couple from North Wales, explain that a lot of their swinging is social. 'I don't have many female friends outside of swinging,' Lisa confesses. 'But, inside swinging, I find it very easy to get along with other women. There doesn't seem to be any jealousy or pettiness when you're with swingers. I suppose a lot of it has to do with the fact that you are all comfortable having sex with each other so, after that handicap has been overcome, there's little that's likely to trouble you. But I think a great part of it is that swingers are naturally better in social situations.'

There are couples who swing and consider it an affirmation of their love for each other. There are couples who swing because their existing sex lives had grown uninspiring and they wanted that additional thrill. Married swingers claim the lifestyle makes the women feel more desirable and can make men more attuned to what is erotic within their relationship. Many singles enjoy a swinging lifestyle because it offers sexual pleasure without the commitment of a relationship. Those involved in alternative relationships (*ménage a trios*, communal living etc.) are adamant that their variation on swinging suits their physical, emotional and economic needs.

But the most obvious reason for swinging, and the most commonly cited by those who participate in the lifestyle, is *purely for the fun*.

Mandy

'. . . if I ever meet a guy with two cocks, I'll probably settle down with him and give up group sex all together . . .'

'My earliest sexual memory is of seeing a porn film. Mum, Dad and Uncle Peter had obviously been up late the night before. Our lounge was never that tidy, but this particular morning it was cluttered with empty beer cans, chocolate wrappers and even a pair of knickers! I was still sleepy. I'd got a glass of milk from the kitchen, and I wandered into the lounge to watch one of my videos as I woke up.'

Mandy is now in her mid-twenties. Her short dark hair frames a face that is pretty despite the harshness of Goth makeup and a complexion as pale as a vampire's.

Speaking with a Scouse accent that conveys confidence and the English epitome of 'street-wise', she rolls a clumsy cigarette as she continues her story. 'I pressed play without checking what was in the VCR. I'd been watching *The Little Mermaid* the night before and I figured it would still be in the machine. But the film that came on wasn't *The Little Mermaid*.'

As soon as she pressed play, the untidy lounge was alive with the sounds of sexual ecstasy. A woman groaned through the pleasure of orgasm. One gruff-voiced male growled for her to take more – the woman moaned in a way that sounded both anguished and delighted – and then a second man was demanding she should beg for 'every mother-fucking inch'.

The screen was alive with pink flesh, obscene in content, gratuitously captured on film, glistening wetly and exploited in frank and uncompromising detail. The shrieks of pleasure and delight were intense, extreme and climactic. The cries were underscored by a backing track of wet slurping sounds and ostentatious sobs for more.

Mandy watched, mesmerised.

'I'd never seen anything like it before. But I knew exactly what it was. The quality of the tape was a little on the shaky side, but it was clear enough that I could see the beautiful redhead in the centre of the screen being screwed by the two men. One of them was sliding his thick cock into her pussy. The other man pushed his cock into her arse. The camera lingered on that scene and showed exactly where all three of them were joined together. Everything looked so glossy, exciting and forbidden. The flesh between her thighs and around her buttocks was wet and shiny. I don't know if I got aroused while I was watching it, or if that came later. But I do know the memory has stayed with me ever since.'

She pauses to light her poorly made cigarette before adding, 'And I also knew, even before Uncle Peter had come rushing down the stairs – turning the VCR off and saying I was a dirty little mare and I shouldn't have been watching "that sort" of movie – I had decided what I wanted out of life. *I wanted to be the woman in the middle.*'

While a great number of childhood vows are forgotten very quickly, Mandy's determination to be the woman in the middle seems to have stayed with her. Her first boyfriend, Barry, was a classmate from school. The pair had allowed their friendship to develop as they attended college together and, after a drunken escape from a dull party, the young couple found themselves naked, embracing and losing their respective virginities.

'It was a disappointment,' Mandy admits. 'It was a big disappointment.'

Barry was a willing and eager lover in bed, but Mandy was quick to notice that he did have shortcomings. 'He only had one penis,' she says giggling. 'I hadn't expected him to have two, and he was OK at using the one that he had. But I'd expected sex to be this great-big-huge-fantastic-dynamic-thrill. And, although it was pretty good, it wasn't as mind-blowing as I knew it would have been if he'd had two penises.'

She laughs and stubs out her cigarette which is already crumbling to a dangerous pile of hot ashes. With disarming honesty, she says, 'I was masturbating regularly by the age of fourteen. I had my own pair of vibrators by the age of sixteen. While a lot of my school friends were out spending their money on cheap cider and crisp packets filled with glue, I spent most of my pocket money buying fresh batteries and Vaseline.'

Because she had such a broad understanding of her own sexual needs, Mandy had no qualms about asking Barry if he could find a friend to join them when they next had sex.

As she lived with her parents at the time, Mandy had to wait until they were out for the evening before she could enjoy her first threesome. Barry had secured the services of his older brother, Graham. It was routine for Mandy's mother and father to go out for a couple of nights over the weekend, and she organised for the two brothers to call on her the following Friday.

Shaking with arousal, spending the day dizzy from a constant buzz of anticipation, Mandy was grinning like a lunatic when the pair arrived within ten minutes of her parents leaving the house. She discovered later that the brothers had been watching from a nearby street corner and were waiting for them to leave.

Graham brought cider. Barry brought a pack of cigarettes. And the three of them retired to the same lounge where Mandy first caught a glimpse of a pornographic video when she had been expecting to watch *The Little Mermaid*.

She puts loud music on the stereo, takes a swig from the bottle of Diamond White and regards Graham warily. Barry hands round the cigarettes. Graham is Barry's senior by little more than a year but he holds himself as though the age difference is far greater. Lounging arrogantly on her parents' settee, gripping the Diamond White and the cigarette as though he is a veteran of such adult accoutrements, he sneers at Mandy. 'Bazzer sez you wanted me to give you a hand with somefink.'

Meeting his gaze, Mandy says, 'Yeah. But it's not your hand I want.' She is wearing a short skirt. Standing up, hitching the skirt to show him the damp crotch of her white cotton knickers, she says, 'Do you think you can help me?'

The effect is instantaneous. A bulge appears at the front of Graham's jeans in the same moment that one sprouts at Barry's. Graham reaches up for her and Barry joins them both on the settee. Mandy's clothes are tugged from her body before she can properly release the first erection. Her small breasts are squashed by cool hands and her bare flesh rubs against coarse denim. The pair are touching and stroking, concentrating on her breasts and pussy. The stimulation is strong enough to have her teetering on the brink of climax within seconds. Catching her breath, forcing herself to remember the few precautions she has considered prior to the start of this evening, she moves herself so she can whisper in Graham's ear, 'We do this on the understanding that you tell no one.'

'Yeah, yeah,' he mutters. His concentration is fixed on sucking a breast.

Mandy pushes his face away and glares at him. 'I mean it,' she insists.

It is difficult to pronounce the words. Her arousal is so fierce she can't properly find the breath to speak. Barry is touching between her legs and the excitement leaves her dizzy. His fingers glide easily against the wetness that has tormented her throughout the day. Each time he touches her clitoris, a fresh bolt of arousal shivers through her body. Nevertheless, she presses on and continues to glower at Graham.

'Do this right for me and we can do it regular and often. But tell anyone and it'll never happen again.'

Graham stares at her truculently. 'I said yeah, didn't I?'

Mandy banishes the hostility of the atmosphere by releasing his erection from his pants. Placing her lips around him, sucking gently on his glans, she mumbles her response around his length. 'I'm glad we understand each other.'

And the sex is everything she had anticipated.

The evening progresses quickly. Within moments, both brothers are naked and Mandy is pressed between them. Their erections squirm urgently towards her holes and, because she has spent the day in a torture of anticipation, Mandy's body is receptive to them both. Barry penetrates first, sliding his wide girth inside her anus and stretching the muscle gently open. Dizzied by the pleasure, Mandy is overwhelmed when Graham forces his shaft into the suddenly tight constraints of her pussy.

Two erections fill her. They slide effortlessly in and out of her holes. Each movement creates an incredible surge of friction. Every breath she takes hurtles her closer to the devastating orgasm she knows she will soon enjoy. The sensation of two nubile bodies being so close, and the satisfaction of being penetrated exactly as she had wanted, proves overwhelming.

'It was absolutely everything that I'd ever wanted,' Mandy explains. 'I was being adored by two young studs. I was being filled exactly as I wanted to be filled. And the orgasm was better than anything you can get from two cheap vibrators and a tub of Vaseline. I'd always known it was going to be good. I'd never doubted that it would be wonderful. But I had never thought it would be such a revelation.'

Her orgasm is so strong that she passes out. She regains consciousness to find Barry and Graham close to panicking because they think they've killed her. The scene must have been amusing – and she has recounted it hundreds of times for the entertainment of close friends – but in that moment she realises she has to soothe the brothers and calm the atmosphere. Barry has been on the verge of phoning an ambulance and Graham is making plans to dispose of her body.

Assuring them that she is OK, encouraging them to finish the remainder of the Diamond White and coaxing each of them to settle down, have a cigarette and relax, she eventually notices that the mood of fright and despair has once again moved back to sultry expectation. She is even more surprised when Graham kisses her cheek and asks softly if she feels sufficiently recovered to 'do it again'.

'It was even better the second time,' she says, giggling. 'After coming once, they both had the stamina I wanted from them. None of us was what you'd call "experienced" but we were quickly learning from each other. Barry was anxious to do whatever he could to please me and Graham was determined to show himself better than his little brother. I was amazed by the effort they put into giving me pleasure and, although I didn't pass out during our second fuck, I did get to heights of pleasure that I'd never been able to reach before.'

Her relationship with Barry and Graham continued until a small rift between the three of them developed into a destructive argument. Barry and Mandy decided they'd had enough of each other and, in an act of mean-mindedness that Mandy found difficult to forgive, one of them spread rumours about her appetites around the college she attended.

Mandy frowns as she recalls the incident. 'There were a couple of nasty nicknames – Dirty Mandy, Double Door Mandy and, naturally, Randy Mandy – but the name calling didn't trouble me too greatly. Most of it was true and when you front people with an honest admission and say, "Yeah? So what?" they back down pretty quickly.' Sighing heavily, she adds, 'But it does wear you down eventually and I pretty much gave up on sex for about a year or two after that. I was nearly nineteen before Alec, one of my tutors from college, asked me if I fancied going with him to a party. I don't think I would have accepted the invitation except for the fact that he added: *it was a swingers' party.* That might have been enough to guarantee me going with him but Alec described the sorts of things that were going to happen. And, when he mentioned the playroom, I don't think anything would have kept me away.'

According to Alec's interpretation of the party, the playroom was where the most sex always happened. Four or more double beds were supposed to be strapped together. A vast sheet was spread over them and then hidden beneath a writhing mass of naked fucking adults. According to Alec, hundreds of couples entered the playroom each evening and they simply fucked whomever they found in there. Any woman lying on the bed could expect to find herself being taken by man after man and enjoying so many multiple penetrations she would think her body had grown new holes.

Alec's language was coarse and his description was vulgar. He whispered the words to her, even though they were alone at the time and away from the risk of being overheard. And he painted exactly the right word picture to make Mandy desperate to attend the swingers' party.

She accepted the invitation and agreed to travel with him that weekend to her first ever swingers' party.

After meeting the hosts, Bill and Beverley, Mandy and Alec don togas and try to get into the party atmosphere. The journey to the party has been a long one and, while they are both tired, neither of them wants to miss a moment of the fun.

'Alec and his wife were swingers,' Mandy explains. 'Until she decided it wasn't for her. They were still married when he invited me to the party and, according to Alec, she had no problems with him continuing to enjoy swinging if it still appealed to him. Consequently, he'd asked me to go as his ticket to Bill and Beverley's party.' (A 'ticket', she explains later, is any willing woman who accompanies an unattached male wishing to attend a swingers' party.)

The house is brightly lit with refreshments freely available. Couples, triples and quartets play easily together, flaunting their nudity and carefree intimacy. Daunted by the whole experience, and betraying her Liverpudlian origins with every syllable, Mandy begins to feel as though she might be out of her element amongst the crowd of sophisticated and experienced swingers.

She has not been at the party for more than five minutes before she has seen two naked women kissing each other. She has watched a man enjoying a blowjob from one woman as he licks the anus of another. And she has watched a submissive male trying to eat grape after grape from the pussy of a dominant female. The openness of the participants' sexualities is staggering.

Mandy's Gothic makeup draws a pleasing amount of positive attention. And, after a fraught half-hour where she wonders if she has made a mistake, her initial doubts and reservations have all but vanished.

'Where's the playroom?' she eventually asks Alec.

Alec shrugs. 'I'm sure we'll find it before the end of the night.' He laughs. 'I've heard it doesn't get busy in there until much later on. Why don't you come and join me in the games' room?'

Reluctant, but not yet ready to relinquish the comfort of being in the presence of the only person she really knows there, Mandy follows Alec down the cellar steps to a brightly lit underground haven. A pool table sits in the centre of the room surrounded by four laughing couples all dressed in togas. Mandy and Alec's arrival is greeted by a hearty cheer and someone shouts, 'Great! We've got another pair to play with.'

Encouraged to join the others, with Alec leading her eagerly into the group, Mandy is treated to a blindfold game where she is kissed, touched and fondled by strangers and then has to guess who was doing what to her. Her toga is taken from her but the nudity doesn't cause any consternation. Lips move against her breasts, mouth, throat, buttocks and pussy. Unseen hands stroke her legs and hips. The stimulation borders on being absolute. Her last qualms are put aside as she gives herself over to the mood of easy familiarity. She cheerfully loses one game, and then another, before going on to help with teasing the next player.

Someone brings down a tray of drinks and nibbles from the party above. Another couple join them and the blindfold game is started afresh.

And Mandy and Alec spend a happy couple of hours playing in the games' room.

'I've never experienced anything so erotic in my life. I was being kissed by women and I was returning those kisses. It had never crossed my mind before to think about eating pussy but I tasted my first one at that party and I could have happily licked it for the remainder of the evening.'

Alec remains attentive to Mandy's needs but it is clear that he is spending some of his time at the party trying to catch up with acquaintances who he would otherwise not see now his wife has withdrawn from swinging. And, while the blindfold game is erotic and stimulating, Mandy remembers that she came to the party for far more than mere titillation. Yet, each time she reminds Alec that she wants to find the playroom, he finds an excuse to delay leading her up there.

She has sex at the party – twice with Alec and once with a dark-skinned girl who calls herself Amy – but the opportunity to find the playroom eludes her. By the time Bill and Beverley are encouraging their guests to leave, Mandy suffers a peculiar feeling of satisfaction intermingled with immense disappointment.

The only thing that stops her from declaring the evening a failure is Alec's promise that, the next time they both attend a swingers' party, he will make sure she gets to spend some time in the playroom.

'The party also acted as a kick up the backside for me,' she says and grins. 'I'd spent two years ignoring my sexual desires, repressing urges when they came along, and doing nothing about my body's need for stimulation and satisfaction. After tasting pussy for the first time, after playing the silly blindfold game – which was like the most surreal kind of foreplay – and after getting screwed by Alec while a crowd of people watched, encouraged and fondled, I was ready to get back on with having a sex life.'

Sighing, pursing her lips to express mild frustration, she says, 'The only problem was Alec never got round to making a second invitation. I was constantly calling him, lurking around the college halls and asking if he had plans to visit Beverley and Bill again, but he was really evasive. I found out later that his wife hadn't been too happy about him continuing to swing once she'd dropped out of the lifestyle. But, rather than being upfront about that, he just kept stalling me. He said Bill and Beverley only held their parties once a month, which was probably true. But he then said he had plans that conflicted with the next party. And the one after that. Then he came up with a whole bunch of other excuses that just got weaker and more pathetic. Eventually, I figured he wasn't going to issue another invitation and I gave up on him.'

But, now that she knew what she wanted, Mandy was determined to get to a playroom through her own endeavours. Alec had driven them to the party without discussing its location, and so she had no way of contacting the couple to ask if they would allow her to attend without him. From the conversations she remembered at the party, and from her own research into swinging afterwards, she knew that single males had difficulty getting through the closed doors of a party but single females were usually welcome. But, without any way of contacting them, Mandy knew she was going to have to find some other venue to realise her ambitions.

Surfing the net at the college's internet café, she found a couple of websites that included contact details for swingers. The thought of submitting an advert crossed her mind but she decided against that idea. More interested in gaining an invitation for a party (with a playroom) than trying to select suitable partners, Mandy sent short queries to a handful of advertisers and explained her needs in embarrassingly frank detail.

She had received three responses by the end of the day. One of them was an invitation to attend a party with a playroom.

For some reason that she can't understand, Mandy is more apprehensive attending her second party than she had been for her first. Regardless of this anxiety, she takes a short train journey from Merseyside to the neighbouring county of Cheshire. And, by the time she has taken a taxi and is approaching the strange front door of a semidetached house in a quiet suburb, her apprehension is close to making her ill.

Nevertheless, adamant that she won't back out now that she is so close to realising her ambition, Mandy pulls on the last reserves of her courage and rings the doorbell.

Karen is an attractive woman, twenty years older than Mandy and dressed in trendy fishnets and a long black T-shirt. Like Mandy, she is wearing heavy Goth makeup that accentuates large expressive eyes and a wan porcelain complexion.

Mandy stammers a greeting and explains she is there for the party.

'You're the internet girl?'

Mandy nods.

The woman kisses her warmly and welcomes her inside. 'You wanted to spend some time in a playroom?'

Mandy nods again, now too embarrassed to speak and not sure how to overcome her sudden shyness. The hostess is clearly used to putting new guests at their ease and slips an arm through Mandy's. 'I'll get you settled in the playroom soon enough,' Karen promises. 'But you look like you could use a drink and a couple of minutes to catch your breath before you start playing.'

Grateful, and almost shaking with relief, Mandy relaxes in the woman's company and feels her anxiety fading away.

The party is already happening as she is led through a hall, past a pair of rooms and back towards a clean modern kitchen. Glancing at everything as she walks through the house, Mandy catches sight of smoky rooms filled with half-naked couples. The images remind her of pornographic videos and ignite her thrill of arousal.

In the kitchen, Mandy sees a pretty blonde, near to her own age, kneeling on the floor of the kitchen and sucking on a burly man's erection. The blonde waves to Mandy and the hostess without moving her mouth from the cock she is working on.

'This is Donna, my daughter,' Karen explains blithely. 'She's the one who organises the parties.'

Continuing to settle Mandy into the party atmosphere, the hostess pours Mandy a cup of tea and gets her to sit at the kitchen table and relax. Donna continues to suck a climax from the burly man before finishing him off and promising to see him later in the evening.

Mandy watches the scene with a mixture of excitement, amazement and arousal.

Although it isn't housed in the same affluent surroundings as the first swingers' party that she attended, Mandy is still impressed by the efforts that have been made by Donna and Karen to make the place comfortable for recreational sex. Couples, triples and foursomes occasionally stumble into the kitchen as Mandy and Karen drink their cups of tea. The other guests are all in various stages of undress and stimulation and their cheerful greetings make Mandy feel properly welcome and wanted.

Intrigued by the relationship that allows the hostess to have her daughter attend and organise a swingers' party, Mandy finds herself bonding with Donna and Karen very quickly. They are open about their needs; neither of them is embarrassed that the other knows of their sexuality, and they don't understand why so many find their mutual involvement in swinging to be such a surprise. They quickly dispel any suggestion of incest and point out that neither of them has a steady man in their life. Swinging parties seemed like a suitable way forwards for both of them and they embrace the lifestyle for giving them what they need when they need it. Their argument is valid and coherent and makes Mandy relax even more in their company. Having accepted the women as genuine friends, she is then delighted when the mother and daughter ask her if she is ready to visit the playroom that she so desperately wanted to attend. Donna takes her left arm and Karen takes her right and the pair escort Mandy up the stairs. And then she is on the verge of stepping inside the playroom.

Alec's vulgar word picture had not done the experience justice. Only two large beds are tied together in this house but their combined size overwhelms the room's available floor space. Lit by the sultry glow of a red light bulb, the scene inside the playroom is like something from an orgasmic vision. Everywhere Mandy turns there is naked flesh. There are so many bare bodies exposed to her that she discovers it doesn't matter whether she is staring at naked men or naked women. Backsides, buttocks, breasts and bodies wriggle together on the bed in a torrid undulation. Gasps, grunts, groans and giggles combine with cries of ecstasy and elation. The scents of feminine musk, masculine sweat and a million more perfumes assail her as she catches one excited breath after another.

She notices that some of the women wear stockings. But they are only a small minority. The few bras and panties Mandy sees are either lying forgotten on the floor or being torn away from bodies to expose more bare flesh.

Donna asks, 'Are you having doubts?'

Before Mandy can reply Karen tells her daughter, 'She's not having doubts. She just doesn't know where to begin.'

And, as she smiles at that reply, Mandy realises Karen has read her mood with frightening precision. No longer hesitant, determined to enjoy the room and all the pleasures it will have for her, Mandy quickly undresses, climbs on to the bed and presses her bare body between two writhing figures.

Two hours later, staggering from the bed in a haze of weak and giddy euphoria, Mandy realises she has achieved her ambition: she has found the thrill she always wanted.

When she later finds Donna and Karen in the kitchen together, Mandy knows that their invitation for her to come to their next party marks the beginning of a long-lasting friendship that she is certain to enjoy.

'I always said, if I ever meet a guy with two cocks, I'll probably settle down with him and give up group sex all together,' Mandy says cheerfully. 'But, Donna and Karen say, if I ever found a guy who's got two cocks, I'd still end up asking him if he's got a friend who might want to join us.' She grins and starts to roll another cigarette. 'I don't know if they're right. But I do know I'm finding exactly what I want at their parties.'

Norman & Olivia
'Married men try harder...'

The atmosphere in the office is incredible. While the humdrum drone of the day begins in every other grey cubicle, Olivia can feel electric tension throbbing in the air around her. The prospect of excitement tingles through her body and she feels bright and alive with daring. Even though James is whispering in her ear, his words falling warm against the side of her neck, her thoughts are with Norman. Even though James has his hand on her shoulder, his thumb stroking slowly down towards the swell of her breast, she can only think about how her husband will respond when she relates the details of this incident back to him. Admittedly, it will be a similar account of events to the one she gave him yesterday evening – James is making advances to her now on a daily basis – but Olivia is happy to be the object of his desire and use that to stimulate her husband's vicarious interest.

'Someone will see,' she tells James.

Despite the words she makes no attempt to stop him. And James is clearly unperturbed by the prospect of discovery. His finger lingers against the front of her blouse. She can feel the warmth of his hand frustratingly close to her nipple.

The bead of flesh stands hard for him. The thrill of taking her flirting this far is enough to turn the crotch of Olivia's panties damp.

'Should we continue this over lunch at the Hansom?' James suggests.

She gasps, shocked, shakes her head and lowers her voice to a whisper. 'A pub lunch is too risky.' She glances at the walls of her cubicle, indicating the other admin staff who share the office. Those few who have started the day early are currently isolated in their own confined worlds but there is nothing to stop anyone from peering into Olivia's workspace, covertly listening from the other side of a partition, or bursting into her booth and pausing, unannounced, by her desk. 'Someone would see us at the pub. There'd be talk,' she explains urgently.

Those final three words are enough to remind James that neither of them wants to incur the nuisance of rumours. 'Do you want me to book the boardroom for our lunch?' James offers.

He has dared to move his fingers lower. He is now stroking the shape of her rigid nipple through the fabric of her blouse. She expected him to flirt with her today and, consequently, Olivia is not wearing a bra. The jacket of her plum suit is open to reveal her white silk blouse. The flimsy fabric is all that separates his fingers from the flesh of her breast. She presses her thighs tight together and trembles in her seat. Because he is standing, she finds herself on eye level with the bulge at the front of his pants. The office is not really a place where she expects to feel or observe excitement and, noticing James's condition, Olivia understands his need for her is as strong as her need for him. Her mouth is dry and it hurts when she tries to swallow. The temptation to touch him makes her ache. She reminds herself to tell Norman about this moment when they are together again in the evening. With a confident knowledge of her husband's tastes and responses, she feels sure that a word painting of this image will have him in an agony of climactic pleasure.

'You think we should meet in one of the boardrooms?' Olivia asks coyly. 'What for?'

'It would give us the chance to continue this privately.'

She considers the suggestion, adoring the flush of arousal that now engulfs her, and contemplating all the things they could do in the privacy of one of the office complex's boardrooms. The wetness between her thighs grows more copious. Her nipples now stand hard and obvious. On an impulse, she strokes the back of her hand against the front of James's pants. The bulge trembles as her knuckles glance against its thickness. James bites back a gasp of excitement.

'Would it be discreet?' Olivia asks.

'No one goes near the boardroom if they think the senior management are in a meeting.'

Chewing her lower lip, trying to present a cool façade and suspecting that she is failing miserably, Olivia asks, 'Can I call you and give you my decision in half an hour?' Her heart hammers in her chest. She believes her attempts to look studied and thoughtful are as transparent as the anti-glare screen on her CRT monitor.

'Send me an email to confirm,' James decides.

He steps quickly back as one of the colleagues from Olivia's team appears in the shared cubicle. Absently fastening his jacket, casually concealing his arousal, he wishes the colleague a good morning, bids Olivia a perfunctory farewell and then disappears.

Olivia immediately phones Norman. Her hands are shaking as she holds the handset against her ear and, twice, she presses the wrong number on her phone's keypad. Eventually, she gets through to him and is relieved to hear the steadying influence of his voice. 'I can't make our lunch date today,' she begins. 'James wants me in the boardroom.'

It had been a struggle to remain calm when she was alone with James but, hearing her husband's excited response, Olivia comes close to giddiness as the heat blossoms through her loins. She keeps the handset pressed tight against her ear, fearful that Norman's shrieks of enthusiasm might be overheard. Her colleague is close enough to hear his louder outbursts and Olivia struggles to remain composed and discreet.

'You don't have any problems with that arrangement, do you?' Olivia asks Norman. She wants to blush when she hears his response. Artfully, she says, 'I'll leave you to handle that on your own. You can fill me in when I get back tonight.'

Not daring to risk any more double entendres, anxious that she might give her secret away if she continues, Olivia reminds her husband that she loves him and then hangs up the phone.

She then sends James an email to confirm their boardroom meeting. Trying to keep the communication simple and inoffensive she writes, *James, just a short line to confirm I can make myself available in the boardroom this lunchtime if you still want me. Olivia.*

At the age of 54, and with a Rubenesque figure that fits comfortably in a size 18, Olivia did not really think her colleague would suspect her of doing anything untoward with James. Without self-deprecation, she admits that her workmates consider her to be fat, plain and bordering on the asexual. But, since her husband encouraged her to start swinging, Olivia firmly believes that there is no other woman in the world, and certainly not in her office building, who has ever felt sexier, more desirable or more erotic.

The hours pass with an unbearable slowness as she waits for the clock to reach noon. The work on her desk remains static and, whenever she takes a telephone call, she mumbles an apology and promises each caller she will get back to them as soon as she has the time to devote her full concentration to their query.

At ten o'clock, James sends an email to confirm that he has booked the executive boardroom from twelve to two. He can even organise for them to have a light lunch shipped up from catering if she's hungry.

Olivia's heart races as she reads the bland message. She writhes restlessly on her seat and then forces herself to sit still for fear that her closest workmate might notice her agitation.

'We haven't always been swingers,' Olivia explains. 'Our sex life had been normal and uneventful until I reached the menopause. Around that time, I put on a lot of weight and then it dried up completely.' She makes the comment without a smile and it is difficult to tell if she has a wry sense of humour or an unusually apt way of making a point.

Continuing, Olivia says, 'Norman kept trying to remind me that he found me attractive but I couldn't see past the mirror image of a fat old woman. When he bought me presents of lingerie and rude toys, I thought he was going soft in the head. I couldn't understand why he was pretending to find me desirable and, eventually, I said as much.' She laughs and says, 'Norman's response was to take naked pictures of me and post them on the internet.'

Olivia can't honestly say why she allowed Norman to take unclothed photographs of her. The idea seemed harmless enough at the time and, even when he posted them to an internet site (with her identity meticulously concealed), she never questioned his explanation that he was doing it for her benefit. 'I was a little bit unsure of what to expect at first. But, when Norman spent an evening showing me the responses my photographs had received – a lot of flattering remarks and some very bawdy suggestions – I was genuinely thrilled to be found desirable. I was so thrilled that I allowed Norman to take some "more daring" pictures. And they received an even better response than the first set.'

But, while the website postings were helping to rekindle Olivia's arousal, she still couldn't shake the belief that she was basically unattractive and past the age of being sexually active. Dismissing the praise she had received from those surfers who had seen her internet pictures, Olivia didn't think the compliments were genuine. It was after she expressed these reservations to Norman that he told her he believed she was incredibly sexy, and he suggested, if she doubted his opinion, she should try and attract another man. The remark heralded a turning point in their relationship.

'I told him it was the most ridiculous suggestion I'd ever heard,' she says, laughing. 'But he was so serious about the idea I eventually tried it.'

Her explanation glosses over the embarrassment, the hesitation and apprehension that she struggled against before daring to go through with the plan. Throughout their thirty years of marriage, Olivia had never entertained the idea of being with another man. While Norman's suggestion appealed to some part of her, she could think of far more reasons to dismiss the suggestion as foolish, unsuitable and inappropriate. Norman persisted, constantly reminding Olivia that he believed she was desirable and repeatedly insisting that she should take a lover to prove, to herself, that she could still excite men.

When Olivia finally relented, she admits that she didn't think Norman would be proved right. Expecting to suffer the humiliation of an embarrassing rejection, she thought her husband might leave their sex life behind after he had seen her upset at being rebuffed.

Yet, the first time she flirted with another man, Olivia was won over by the genuine pleasure that came from feeling wanted and desired. Even though they did nothing more than kiss and touch intimately, the thrill was greater than she had anticipated. And, from that simple beginning, and with her husband's constant encouragement and approval, she quickly progressed to being bolder and more daring with each new man.

Shortly before noon, James calls Olivia and reminds her they have a luncheon appointment in one of the main boardrooms. The reminder is unnecessary – Olivia has not been able to think of anything else throughout the morning

– but she thanks him and assures him that she will be there. Aware that colleagues might be listening to her conversation, she asks him if she should bring anything.

'Make sure you bring your appetite,' he replies, and then hangs up.

It is a struggle for Olivia to maintain her composure as she makes her way to the meeting. She spends ten minutes in the lavatories, reapplying her makeup and freshening up before heading towards the boardroom. This is not the first time she has taken a lover but the experience always leaves her weak with arousal, nervousness and anticipation.

She worries about every possible thing that can go wrong: the lift might break down on its way up to the third floor, leaving her stranded and unable to make the date; someone might guess what they are doing and inform senior management; James might suddenly be repulsed by the idea of having sex with her and leave her jilted and alone in the boardroom.

All these considerations are brushed from her mind when she finds herself alone in the boardroom with James and a plate of fresh cream cakes. It is a spacious office, large enough to give the paradoxical sense of functional ostentation that is the current vogue amongst successful businesses. A polished teak table dominates the room and is surrounded by elegant minimalist chairs. One wall of polarised windows overlooks the landscaped areas to the west of the office buildings. Another presides over the well-maintained and leafy splendour of the executive car park.

Olivia notices that there is a conference phone in the centre of the room and she wishes she had had the foresight to arrive early and phone home. With the telephone on speaker, Norman would have been able to hear every grunt, groan and gasp as she and James became physically acquainted. Knowing how much he craves a fuller involvement with her when she is swinging, Olivia has to bite her lip to stop herself from asking James if he would mind if she quickly made a call so she can leave the line open.

James locks the door behind Olivia, takes her in his embrace, and then they kiss. He touches her face as their lips meet and Olivia notices that the hand sports a solid gold band on the third finger. When the cool metal touches her cheek, she trembles.

'Married men try harder,' Olivia confides. 'I don't know why that is. Perhaps it's because they're used to disappointing their wives, so they make an extra effort when they're having a fling.' She shrugs the comment away, apologises for her cynicism and explains that she prefers to take married lovers, although she can't pinpoint her preference to one specific reason. 'Married men are more likely to be discreet,' she explains. 'They're usually free from diseases. And they're less likely to think there's more to what we're doing than just sex.'

Her smile is bitter and bordering on the defensive as she adds, 'I don't feel wholly right about sleeping with married men. I do know that I'm encouraging them to be unfaithful. But the chances are they would have been unfaithful with someone else if I hadn't come along. And I know I'm not going to tell anyone. And I know the men I sleep with aren't going to tell their wives – which means it's just a little bit of harmless fun between consenting adults.'

James pulls the blinds closed to ensure their privacy. The boardroom is three floors up but neither of them feels brave enough to court the attention of those in neighbouring buildings or lunching co-workers who might choose to glance up at their window at precisely the right/wrong moment.

Holding Olivia by the hips, James leads her to the pastries. 'What do you fancy?' he asks.

Her answer, she confesses afterwards, is predictable. But it is enough to get them kissing again. And, while they have two hours alone together, they go at each other with the same urgency they would have shown if they only had two minutes together.

Olivia unfastens his pants. James steals a hand inside her blouse. In the same moment that she touches the scalding flesh of his erection, he is stroking the hard nub of her nipple. Their gasps of appreciation are justifiably muted – the boardroom isn't soundproofed and orgiastic cries would run a risk of being overheard – but neither of them is whispering as they assure the other of their need.

Olivia's sex is a hungry mouth that needs to devour James. When he stops teasing her breasts, his fingers slip between her legs and glide easily inside her welcoming pussy. She knows his erection will be thick enough to satisfy her needs and, after his tongue has slipped against her sex lips for a few glorious moments, she is desperate to feel him inside her.

James helps Olivia on to the boardroom table, pushing her skirt up and pulling her thighs apart. The teak groans under her weight and, for an instant, she frets about how they would explain a broken board table to the executive committee. And then James is moving his face back down to the cleft of her sex and the worry of breaking the deceptively sturdy desk is cast from her thoughts.

'No,' Olivia gasps. His tongue is sliding frenziedly against the molten flesh of her pussy lips. She is already wet and aching to have him penetrate her and the idea of suffering any more cunnilingus is more than she can tolerate. Her voice is hoarse with arousal as she gasps again, 'No. Please. Don't.'

James glances up at her, concerned and wondering if, for some bizarre reason, she is now changing her mind about what they will do together. 'But I thought . . .' he begins. His voice trails off when he sees the desperate need in her face.

'Fuck me, James,' she growls. 'No more pussy-kissing. Just fuck me.'

He grins at her and begins to remove his pants. His shirt is already hanging outside the open waistband and Olivia has managed to expose his erection through the fly of his trousers. But, on Olivia's instruction, he steps out of the trousers and climbs between her legs.

'Do you know how long I've waited for this?' he asks.

Olivia laughs huskily and says, 'Probably just as long as me.'

It's the last thing she manages to say before James is urging his thick length between her thighs and into her sex.

'The sex with other men is usually pretty good,' Olivia admits. 'But it's the sex afterwards that I find superior. That's why I do it.'

Norman squeezes her hand and thanks her for the implicit compliment. Considering the affection between the pair, it is clear that their swinging is carried out specifically for the pleasure of each other.

Their time in the boardroom finishes about fifteen minutes before the two hours are up. After being taken across the boardroom table, and brought to a climax that had her biting her fist to mute the exclamations, Olivia peels away James's used condom, stuffs it into her handbag and then proceeds to lick and suck his exposed flesh until he is hard again.

The taste of his semen is invigorating. She normally tries to avoid exchanging bodily fluids when playing with a lover but there is no way she can send James out of the boardroom to clean himself. Also, because it's so rare that she allows herself to taste another man, Olivia always finds the flavour of a new cock to be a powerful and forbidden aphrodisiac.

He is hard again within minutes and eager to carry on where he left off. Olivia continues to suck him for a while longer, delighting in the sensation of his bare erection on her tongue and between her lips. Then she rolls another condom over his shaft and guides him between her thighs.

This time, she straddles James, making sure her large thighs aren't pressing too heavily on his hips and squatting on her haunches to get him deeper inside. Rolling her pelvis back and forth, urging his length to rub hard against the throb of her clitoris, she pushes herself to the brink of another climax as James claws at her breasts and struggles to stave his own ejaculation.

This time, as they both enjoy their orgasms, James and Olivia have to kiss to stop their exclamations from being loud enough to escape the discretion of the boardroom. They end their lunchtime together spent and satisfied. James kisses Olivia, thanks her and then leaves her to the pastries as he goes outside the building to the designated smoking area.

Olivia uses the boardroom's conference telephone to call her cubicle colleague and says she's just finished her meeting and is now going home for the remainder of the day.

When her workmate expresses concern, and asks if there is a problem, Olivia almost giggles hysterically when she demurs that James gave her a lot to think about. The truth of the statement is enough to bring her close to horrified laughter as she realises her thoughts are full of every explicit detail of the afternoon.

After making a quick call to Norman, and telling him she's on her way back home, Olivia flees from the building, gets into her car and drives back to her husband.

Norman says, 'For me, it's the most exciting thing in the world to have Olivia come home flushed from fucking another man. I don't know why it turns me on so much. I think it's because she's had her sexiness reaffirmed. She always seems to carry herself as though she's got a secret or something forbidden that she's slyly proud of. I can't properly define the reason it excites me so much but I do know there's nothing sexier in the world.'

He licks his lips before continuing. 'I would dearly love to watch her with another man,' he admits eventually. 'But, so far, that hasn't happened. I suppose it's difficult enough for someone with Olivia's confidence to actually flirt with other men and find the courage to have sex with them. It's asking a lot to expect her to add a really unsettling kink to the situation by suggesting she should bring her husband along to watch them fuck.'

As soon as she is in the house, Norman is trying to embrace his wife and get details from her. Blushing, acting with a coyness that contrasts harshly with her behaviour of an hour earlier, Olivia says she wants a glass of wine before she tells him anything. A practised tease, Olivia makes Norman pour her the drink and settle himself down at her feet and then slips him morsels of information as she would give titbits to a well-trained pet.

Basking in his position beneath her, Norman begs for more and more details. Olivia patiently takes him through the morning, explaining how James touched her, what he suggested and how excited she felt. And then she tells her husband to stop wanking himself and pay more attention to her. After waiting until he is squirming obediently on the floor, then demanding kisses to her feet, thighs and breasts before she deigns to continue, Olivia only carries on when Norman is doing everything she has told him.

The conversation draws on through an hour of foreplay during which Olivia climaxes three times. Norman does everything she asks: tonguing her sex, replenishing her glass of wine and attentively hanging on her every word. When Olivia says she is hungry, Norman rushes to fix a light salad from the fridge. Each time Olivia says she is thirsty, he replenishes her glass of wine. He dutifully goes through her handbag at Olivia's command, retrieving the spent condoms before depositing them in the kitchen waste bin. Handling the physical remainder of the thin sheath that separated his wife's sex from the erection of her lover, he trembles with raw arousal.

Norman's exhilaration is constant. His enthusiasm to hear every detail and vicariously relive his wife's moment of illicit passion is sincere and without affectation.

And, when Olivia finally allows him to enter her sex, the build-up has been so intense for him the act is over within three torturous thrusts.

Not disappointed by this reaction, clearly delighted that she has been able to inspire her husband with so much excitement, Olivia spends the next half-hour teasing him back to a state of full erection as she touches and kisses him, while sharing more details of her time in the boardroom with James.

The sex is interspersed with more glasses of wine and a light meal, before an early night. They are both physically drained from the day's lovemaking but Olivia has one final remark to make as they slip into bed together and prepare to sleep. 'James asked about seeing me again,' she whispers.

Norman is instantly alert and hanging on her words. His penis had been languishing but, as soon as she mentions seeing James again, the flesh begins to thicken in readiness for her. 'What did you say?'

'I told him I'd love to see him again. But only on one condition.'

'A condition? What condition?'

'If he gets to see me again, I told him that I wanted you in the room at the same time.' She smiles as her husband covers her face with grateful kisses and presses his burgeoning erection against her sex. Anxious that he shouldn't build up his hopes too highly, she adds, 'James hasn't said yes or no yet. He's still thinking about whether or not he can deal with another man being in the room at the same time.'

Not discouraged by this proviso, Norman continues to kiss his wife and thrusts inside her. This time the sex continues for a long uninterrupted hour. They repeatedly change positions, perpetually striving for a greater thrill and a different sensation. When the final climax of the day defeats them both, they drift off to a sleep that is encouraged by equal measures of satisfaction and exhaustion.

And, as they lie happily in each other's arms, it is obvious that both Norman and Olivia know perfectly well why they enjoy swinging.

David & Pamela
'. . . I'd wanted more honesty . . .'

David pushes himself gently inside Margaret.

After two months of illicitly seeing each other, they have progressed to a stage in their relationship where they need something more to sustain the variety and excitement. This is the first time Margaret has allowed him to penetrate her anus and they have agreed to take the development carefully. His penis is larger than her husband's – in length if not in thickness – and David is anxious that this experience should be pleasurable for them both. Slowly, after easing the head of his sheathed glans through her sphincter, he pushes deeper.

Margaret grunts appreciatively beneath him. Her fingers are pulling at her pussy lips and squeezing hard at her clitoris. This sex act is taboo – something she has never done with her husband or any previous lover – and the balance of pain and pleasure mesh uneasily in those first few moments. It is only when arousal sweeps the last of her reservations aside that she pushes herself down to meet his penetration.

She feels warm, lubricated and inviting. Her encouragement comes in impassioned whispers spat from between tightly clenched teeth. Loud music on the stereo nearly covers their mounting cries of pleasure, as they growl at each other with incoherent murmurs of adulation.

And neither of them notices David's wife, Pamela, appear in the doorway. They don't realise she is there until Pamela turns off the music and screeches, 'What the fuck is going on here?'

The answer to her question is made horribly clear when David pulls himself away from Margaret. Pamela is treated to the sight of the woman's momentarily gaping anus. The muscle closes almost as soon as his erection is retrieved from her, but Pamela is left with the lingering image of Margaret's backside opened up after being used by David's cock.

David's adultery with Margaret was not a complete shock to Pamela. She had returned early to their home and entered quietly because she suspected something was amiss. But she had only expected to find the pair kissing. Catching the pair entangled in 'that most forbidden act' did come as an unpleasant surprise. And the memory of seeing such gross intimacy was impossible to shake.

Their argument began while Margaret dressed and fled. Pamela regaled her with a volley of abuse that she felt justified in delivering. *Margaret was a whore; a married woman covertly fucking someone else's man; a filthy bitch who took it up the arse.*

Pamela hurled the insults despite David's pleas that she should calm down, and didn't stop until Margaret had rushed half-dressed from the house in a tearful search for a taxi home. And then David and Pamela began to argue.

The quarrel continued into the night; the word divorce was bandied around frequently and between a lot of expletives; and it wasn't until the early hours of the morning that David and Pamela resolved to save their marriage and settle the differences that had driven them to this situation.

Reflecting on the incident, they both concur that the conclusion of the conversation was a simple recipe for success: they needed to be more honest with each other.

'Pamela said she was more hurt by the fact that I'd deceived her rather than the fact that she'd caught me having sex with Margaret.' David blushes, as he admits, 'I can understand that. I'd felt pretty bad about going behind her back. But our relationship had been a fairly normal one up to that point. I don't know anyone in a normal relationship who can turn to his wife and say, "I fancy fucking Margaret, and maybe slipping it up her arse. You don't have any problems with that, do you, sweetheart?"'

Neither of them fancied the idea of counselling. The prospect of dredging up their private lives in front of an unknown 'expert' was something they were both anxious to avoid. They considered a variety of options that included pretending nothing had happened, David having psycho-therapy and even trying for another child. In amongst the wide range of solutions they discussed, they unexpectedly found themselves returning to the idea of swinging.

David honestly admits that swinging seemed less like a solution to their problem and more like a surreal bonus prize for being caught in an act of adultery. But he seriously thought it might be a solution to the problems affecting their marriage.

Pamela was struggling to recover from the breach of trust and desperately wanted to inject more honesty into their relationship. She had read a couple of articles on the subject of swinging and remembered someone saying that the levels of honesty between swinging couples were far greater than those between those who didn't swing. The lifestyle made sense to her – in an open relationship, there would be no need for either of them to hide any aspect of what they were doing – and she and David decided, paradoxically, that having other lovers might be what was needed to keep their marriage together. Swinging was an alternative that would allow David the extramarital liaisons he clearly craved, while assuring Pamela of the honesty that she believed their relationship needed.

'I'd never had any particular interest in swinging before,' Pamela admits. 'But I'd always thought it was better for a couple to know what their partners were doing, rather than one of them come home early one night and find her husband buggering his best friend's wife.'

David adds, 'I had heard people say that swinging was more of an addition to a healthy relationship rather than a tonic for one that was failing. But I knew our relationship wasn't failing. Pamela and I were still good together. I was just responsible for making a silly mistake.'

He organised their first night with another couple within the month.

John and Carol are similar in age and status to David and Pamela. It is not their first time swinging but they don't class themselves as experienced. After meeting up in a local pub – Carol looking resplendent in a short skirt and low-cut top, John smelling clean and desirable with an Armani fragrance to match his suit – the two couples quickly bridge the nervousness of the situation. Pamela's laughter sounds genuine, David's warm humour has them all chuckling and there is an electric charge to the atmosphere when the foursome realise they are going to spend the night together.

John offers to go to the bar to get fresh drinks and Pamela asks if he wants her to go with him and help. Left alone, David and Carol move closer and begin to touch each other in a more familiar manner.

His arm moves around her waist. She places a hand on his knee. Pressing her face close to his ear, whispering to make the revelation more discreet, Carol says, 'I think my husband wants to fuck your wife.'

The remark plunges a hot spike of excitement through David's stomach. He suddenly wishes John and Pamela would hurry back: not because he wants to see either of them in any great hurry but because he needs the drink they are fetching.

'Would you object to your husband fucking my wife?' David asks softly.

Carol shakes her head. 'I'd like to watch.' She grins eagerly as her hand slips from his knee and moves over the throbbing bulge in his lap. 'And, once we've watched them,' she continues, 'I'd like them to watch you and me so we can show them how it's properly done.'

The atmosphere of the smoky pub is no longer around them. David is thrilled by the excitement of what they are doing and what they are going to do. He leans into a kiss from Carol and she responds with urgent haste. Their mouths are still locked together when John and Pamela return to their table.

'The irony of the whole thing was, I'd suggested we try swinging so that we could be more honest,' Pamela confides. 'But with swinging comes this huge burden of a secret that you've got to keep from other people by constantly lying. Isn't that just a truly perfect irony?' She laughs, a rare but engaging sound, and quotes conversations she has used to cover up her participation in swinging.

'Where are you going this weekend?'

'Oh! We're just going to see friends.'

'Don't your friends want you to bring the kids along now and again?'

'They're not really into kids. And you know how much the kids enjoy staying with you.'

Pamela's smile tightens and the expression of good humour disappears from her eyes.

'What did you get up to this weekend?'

'Nothing much. We just spent a little time with some close friends.'

'Is that all you got up to? You look really smug and contented. What have you been doing?'

'Nothing. I've told you. Nothing.'

Sighing wearily she explains, 'I'd wanted more honesty. And, while I got that from David, I also got lumbered with having to tell lies to my friends and family. The strain quickly made me miserable and I began to wonder if I'd made a truly foolish mistake because having to lie wasn't the only thing I didn't like about swinging.'

* * *

Later, in private, watching John with Pamela, David feels a surge of arousal that is strong enough to make him shake. Her naked body lies beneath John, her bare legs are wrapped around John's waist, and she pushes her pelvis up to meet each thrust. David is in the perfect position to see John's sheathed shaft enter Pamela. The slender pink lips engulf John's erection. David avidly watches another man enter his wife's sex. He inhales the musky scent of her arousal, knowing it has been inspired by someone else. And he hears her gasp with a sexual pleasure that has not been caused by his attention. The moment is electric and spellbinding and a hundred and one other clichés that all sum up his over-whelming excitement. Seeing the pair kiss, watching Pamela throw herself into the act with a hunger she has not shown him in a long time, he feels sure their dormant desires will soon be rekindled to the frenzied lust they had once shared. In his excitement, he almost forgets that he is supposed to be pleasuring Carol. Mumbling an apology, he places his erection between her legs and slides inside her.

Watching David with Carol, Pamela feels as though she is going to vomit. Attractive, cheerful and blessed with a perfect figure, Carol rides David with a vigour that Pamela knows she could never match. His features are animated with a strength of arousal she cannot recall seeing on his face before. The sight of him embracing the woman reminds her of the night she caught David pushing his cock deep into Margaret's backside.

Her position allows her a glimpse of the penetration. And, while she is touched by a finger of excitement at the sight of her husband's shaft pushing into Carol's smoothly shaved pussy, Pamela finds herself remembering how Margaret's anus had looked when David hurriedly withdrew from her rear.

Her need to vomit is almost too close to avoid. When John closes his mouth over hers in a long and lingering kiss, she has to force herself to respond for fear that she will otherwise just pull herself away and run from the whole nightmarish scene. She has been prepared to fake her orgasm to show willing for this first experience in swinging but she is suddenly fearful that either David, John or Carol will be able to tell the difference between her acting and the genuine article. That worry becomes immaterial when a surge of raw pleasure rushes through her. But the climax is still mostly joyless.

'We went with three or four other couples after that,' David explains.

'I hated it more and more each time,' Pamela admits. 'The true irony of the situation was, I'd wanted more honesty, and I'd got it from David at the expense of my honesty with my family and friends. Then, to make the irony complete, I'd stopped being honest with him. I couldn't tell him how much I hated the swinging. He was enjoying it; we were having open discussions about our responses, and what constituted an erotic experience. And the thought of telling him that I wasn't enjoying the swinging would have made me look like some fickle, shallow, lying hypocrite.'

'So,' David says without rancour, 'instead of telling me that she's unhappy with the situation, Pamela simply ended one of our swinging nights by smashing me over the head with a heavy glass ashtray.' He wears a wry smile as he adds, 'It was around then that I began to suspect things might not be working out as well as I'd hoped.'

On an April night in 2004, David spent a couple of hours in the A&E department of his local hospital, received seven stitches to his scalp and blundered his way through a flimsy excuse for the benefit of the police officers who questioned him about the assault.

'It was an accident. My wife was pretending to hit at me, and her judgement must have been a bit off. She'd had a couple of drinks. We all had. I'm sure there's no need for this matter to be investigated by the police.'

'Is this your wife, sir?

'No. This is Janet. She's a . . . she's a friend. Janet and her husband Jim were with my wife and I when this happened.'

'And can you corroborate your *friend*'s version of events?' the police officer asks Janet.

Janet nods. She is clearly shocked by all that has happened but she has sufficient wits about her to confirm David's story. She makes no mention of the exact details: she and David had been interlocked in the doggy position; David's sheathed erection was sliding gently into her anus; behind them, Pamela had moaned something that sounded like '*not again*'; Janet had felt David turn to see what was happening and then heard him gasp a protest. She had felt the shock of something heavy echoing through her body; that motion came at the same time as she heard the dull thud of two weighty objects colliding; and then he had collapsed, unconscious, on top of her. And the screaming had begun.

'And where is your wife now?' the police officer asks David.

Janet answers, 'My husband is looking after her at her home.'

Pamela says shortly, 'The ultimate irony is, now I'm with another man, what I've done in the past still won't allow me the honesty I always craved. Andy is a good man, and he's told me all about his life experiences so far. But I can't be honest with him and tell him the truth about why David and I separated. He knows I found David with another woman. And I've told him that we tried to make things work for a while after that. But he doesn't know that it was our attempts at swinging that ultimately drove David and I apart.'

Pamela shakes her head and sits back in the lounge's stiff leather settee. This is the same room where she first caught David and Margaret engaged in anal sex and it is clear that she is still not comfortable in the location. Her lower lip trembles as though she is on the verge of tears and her eyes are wide and haunted.

'David has been good about the divorce. I suppose he's been a lot more understanding than many husbands would have been after suffering concussion. I've got the house and, once I've decided whether or not he's a subversive influence, I'll probably let him see the kids again.'

She shakes her head again, suddenly angry, and says, 'Swinging is so much bullshit. I don't really think it works for anyone. It broke up me and David. I'm sure swinging was the reason why Jim and Janet are no longer together. Margaret isn't with her husband since he found out what she'd been doing with David.' Pamela rushes through that final sentence, as though fearful it might be misinterpreted if someone dwells on its meaning for too long. 'And I'd be interested to find out if John and Carol or any of those other swinging couples are still married.'

She stares quietly at the grand piano in the corner of the room and then turns her attention to the recessed ceiling lights that brighten our conversation. When she finally blinks and remembers the point of the conversation, she resumes with the words, 'I know what's in the past is in the past. But, knowing how David responded to me with another man, I worry Andy will respond the same way if I tell him about that part of our lives.' Frowning bitterly, she adds, 'And, if Andy ever suggested swinging, I don't think I would be able to trust him ever again. That would definitely spell the beginning of the end for us.'

Janet squeezes David's hand and says, 'With or without swinging, I think David and Pamela's marriage would have come to an end within that year. In one way, I'm sorry that they tried swinging because it's clearly upset Pamela. But, in a positive light, it's given David and me a chance to meet and be together that we wouldn't have had if they hadn't tried the lifestyle.' She kisses him with genuine affection and, with a show of maternal caring, wipes tears from the corners of his eyes. 'When you look at it in a positive light,' she adds tenderly, 'you begin to realise that things haven't turned out quite so bad.'

Glancing around the shabby apartment they share, absently fingering the side of his head, as though his scar is uncomfortable, David forces himself to smile in agreement. 'Yes,' he says firmly. 'You begin to realise things haven't turned out quite so bad.'

And, although the couple are no longer swinging as they try to start their own family, they are both adamant that, one day, they will be having their fun with other couples.

HOW DO YOU SWING?

The 60s and 70s image of swingers – wife-swapping parties where wives randomly select car keys from a bowl, and spend the evening with the gentleman associated with the vehicle – is the only enduring stereotype to taint the image of those involved in the lifestyle.

Some swingers continue to play games of random selection at parties. Playing cards is a popular method, leaving the choice of partner to chance rather than personal selection. Car keys still feature at some retro parties while more modern elements such as mobile phones, business cards and Post-it notes have all been exploited in one form or another.

But these games are only played at the more organised parties and, even then, the 'randomness' is subject to stringent rules of pre-selection prior to participation. Consequently, it is not surprising to note that the majority of swingers now favour recreational sex with someone they find attractive and have personally selected rather than someone thrown into their arms by chance.

Swapping is probably one of the most common methods of swinging. This is at its most simplified when two couples simply swap partners and have sex before returning to their regular partners. Variations on this theme can include mutual masturbation, oral sex instead of penetration, the four having sex in the same room, the two women having sex together while the husbands/boyfriends watch, or whatever the four have previously agreed would be their ideal outcome for the evening. (NB. For safety, and until they are past the nerves of their first few encounters, many experienced couples advocate same-room swinging for those who are new to the lifestyle.)

Soft swinging is the clinical term for intimacy between existing partners while others are present in the same room. This can range from kissing and touching, right up to extreme exhibitionism and penetrative sex. But, with soft swinging, penetration only ever occurs between existing partners.

Camming is a contemporary variation on soft swinging and involves the current vogue for using webcams. This alternative to cyber-sex allows couples and singles to enjoy a discreet sexual liaison through the internet. Using webcams, microphones, chatroom software and sufficient computer knowledge to keep their identity private, they are able to communicate, watch and encourage each other through various stages of masturbation. This twenty-first-century version of soft swinging is an ideal meeting place for voyeurs and exhibitionists. In some chatrooms, it is not uncommon to find proud singles and couples happily broadcasting their naked images to a hundred or more voyeurs. Those cammers less inclined to such public displays retreat to the sanctuary of private chatrooms for more intimate times together.

Obviously, as mentioned elsewhere in this book, there are also parties and clubs and those spontaneous encounters that frequently prove serendipitous to the needs of wannabe swingers.

Adverts for swingers can be found and placed in a variety of magazines that include *Forum*, *Desire* and *Contacts*, as well as the majority of adult magazines and many local newspapers.

Alternatively, and fast becoming the preferred method of communication for swingers today because of its ease, convenience and the speed of responses, the internet hosts a huge range of sites for swingers that include www.wifelovers.com, www.loungeparties.com and www.local swingers.co.uk, among too many others to mention.

The lexicon of terminology involved (*CPL, 35M, 28F(AC/DC) seek similar or bi-fem for BDSM and ultimate*) can usually be translated by the helpful glossaries provided by most internet sites and the sidebars available in the more thoughtful magazines.

And, after deciding how to make initial contact and settling on a preferred method of swinging, the only remaining requirements are a mutual desire and a great deal of courage.

The photographer behind the Diverse Publications title, *My Wife and Her Lovers* (an erotic photo-journal capturing the couple's journey into swinging) says, 'It amazed us how many people thought it was a good idea, until the time came to meet. We were stood up loads of times! That showed us that many people have fantasies but most are frightened to fulfil them.'

It is repeatedly stressed that those couples who lose their nerve at the last moment are the bane of experienced swingers. Whether it's soft swinging, dogging, visiting clubs, parties, orgies or simply meeting a likeminded couple, the most important requirement is having the bravery to take that first step.

Sonia & Roger
'I came so hard on his face . . .'

S onia had decided how the evening would progress before they went out. Dressed in a short black skirt, high heels and a white top, she mentally described the outfit as 'tarty' before presenting herself to Roger. The skirt showed off more leg than she normally dared to reveal, stopping just after the curve of her modest buttocks. The top was tight and sheer, making it obvious she was braless beneath. The thin fabric darkened over the circles of her areolae and her nipples bulged noticeably. Willowy in stature, with blonde curls framing an elfin face, Sonia thought the reflection in her bedroom mirror looked nothing like the woman she was used to seeing there.

Unaware of what she was planning, Roger nodded tacit approval and assured his wife she looked OK, before leading the way to the local working men's club. It was only a short walk from their terraced home, the summer evening clement enough so that neither of them needed a jacket, and they arrived to find the bar already busy with friends and neighbours sharing drinks and conversations.

'You look very nice this evening,' John told Sonia. John was one of Roger's closest friends and he made the declaration as he brought drinks for the three of them. Flattery wasn't usually in his nature and Sonia thought her 'tarty' outfit must have been eye-catching to elicit his compliment. She thanked him for the drink, took a sip of lager to steady her nerves and proceeded to tell him about the latest DVD she and Roger had added to their collection. 'You'd love it,' she gushed. 'It's totally filthy.'

He raised an eyebrow.

Dropping easily into the thread of the conversation, Roger nodded confirmation of this verdict.

One aspect of their friendship involved a mutual appreciation of adult movies. John spent a lot of time travelling throughout Europe and seemed able to find foreign titles that were far more adventurous and explicit than anything Roger or Sonia could usually get hold of in South Wales. But they shared their discoveries and were always eager to mention the stronger elements to watch out for in each film.

Roger had received the most recent title for their collection as an unexpected gift from his brother on holiday. Because its content was very strong, Sonia thought it compared favourably with the titles John had previously lent to them. The penetration shots were graphic; the cast were attractive and desirable; and the sex scenes were filmed in leering and gratuitous detail.

'It's got a real slutty blonde as the main girl,' Sonia explained. She gave John a meaningful glance and added, 'I know you like real slutty blondes.'

He smiled.

'You'll have to borrow it one night,' Roger told him.

'I must,' John agreed.

'You don't have to borrow it,' Sonia said quickly.

She could feel Roger studying her warily as she spoke. Considering the fantasies they'd recently confessed to each other, she guessed he had an idea what she was plotting. But he said nothing.

'When we've finished here, you could come round and watch it at ours,' Sonia suggested.

She held her breath once she'd spoken, wondering if the words sounded contrived or if the tone of her voice had given away her plans. Roger's wary expression remained pointed in her direction, and Sonia guessed he knew what she wanted. But it was John who she watched as she waited for his response.

He took another sip at his lager and shook his head. 'I can't tonight,' he apologised. 'I'm entertaining guests.' He nodded in the direction of an adjacent table and Sonia saw two strangers drinking pints and chatting together.

John explained they were colleagues – guys he had previously met while working overseas – and they were staying at his home so the three of them could make the weekend journey together to the same work site in Germany for a Monday-morning start.

'I'll have to call round when I'm next back,' John said. With a rueful glance at his colleagues he added, 'And when I don't have Joseph and Richard with me.'

Sonia made the change to her plans without pausing to fret about the consequences. Afterwards, she realised it was a huge decision but at the time it seemed only natural to say, 'You can bring them with you, if you like.'

Roger gave her a doubtful glance.

'Are you sure?' John asked. He spoke with an innocence that was maddening and Sonia longed to know if he understood what she was subtly suggesting, or if he really did think the invitation she had made was simply to watch a late-night showing of a risqué movie.

She snatched a big gulp from her pint and nodded. 'The more the merrier,' she assured him.

Listening to the words, she silently marvelled at her own daring and wondered if Roger would allow the evening to progress the way she hoped. The thrill of sexual arousal was already enough to make her feel weak. She could feel her nipples pressing against the tight polyester of her top. The only thing threatening to spoil the night was Sonia's paranoid belief that everyone in the working men's club knew about her scheme.

John invited Joseph and Richard to join them at the table and idly mentioned the movie they would be watching after they'd finished at the club. The pair were enthusiastic and the following couple of hours hurtled past in a whirl of nervous laughter, too many pints and cheerfully lewd conversation. Joseph and Richard turned out to be fun company and Sonia could tell they were attracted to her from the repeated blushes they suffered each time she caught one or the other glancing at her stiff nipples. Her excitement grew stronger as the evening progressed.

When they staggered out of the working men's club, the five of them were still laughing and joking. Sonia knew she had drunk more than her usual limit but the night's cool air sobered her instantly. She had a brief moment of hesitation, nerves plagued her that she might be risking too much, or misjudging the mood of the four men.

Roger held her arm as they walked and she could tell he was trying to slyly whisper some question in her ear. But the others were always too close for them to converse discreetly. By the time she had thought he might be asking about her plans, they were back home. And, as she watched the four men file through her front door, Sonia was suddenly determined that she wouldn't back out.

Roger, John, Richard and Joseph settled themselves in the lounge while Sonia went to the kitchen. Her stomach churned as she dragged tins of beer from the fridge but she steeled herself against the idea of backing out now she had come this far.

Making sure no one could see, confident that she was alone in the kitchen, Sonia removed her panties. Her heart pounded. The crotch of the panties was sodden and she realised she had spent the evening in a state of constant arousal. Blushing at her own boldness, she threw the panties in the laundry and took the beers to the lounge.

Roger sat in his usual seat, close to the lounge door. The TV set was in the opposite corner and John, Joseph and Richard were squeezed together on the settee that nestled against the wall. Their conversation continued unabated as Sonia handed out the cans. She placed her own drink on the coffee table in the centre of the room before going to the modest collection of DVDs and selecting their most recently acquired title.

'Are you sure you boys won't be embarrassed watching this?' she asked, waving the explicit cover of the box so they could see what they were going to watch.

Roger and John laughed. Joseph and Richard exchanged broad grins and shook their heads. After popping the tabs from their cans and taking a swallow, they placed the drinks with feigned nonchalance over their laps and all settled back and allowed Sonia to load the DVD.

'I had my back to the settee,' she said afterwards. 'I could hear the boys were still chatting as I bent over to load the movie. Then the room just went deathly silent. And I knew they were all looking at my pussy. I'm surprised I didn't come there and then.'

Sonia slid the DVD into the player and moved backwards, away from the TV set, as the film began to load. She didn't dare look at any of the men on the settee. Pretending that nothing had happened she sat on the arm of Roger's chair and then reached for her beer can. The atmosphere in the room was so tense she found it difficult to breathe. John, Richard and Joseph were deliberately not looking at her, their gazes fixed intently on the TV screen. Although they each kept their tin of beer in their lap, Sonia could not resist smiling when she saw each of them was trying to hide an erection. That sight was enough to buoy her confidence and assure her that the evening would be a success.

Roger placed his arm around Sonia's waist and pulled her close so he could place a kiss against her cheek. Taking the opportunity to whisper in her ear he asked, 'What are you planning?'

'Planning?' she murmured. Guessing that he already knew the answer, she returned his kiss and said, 'I'm not planning anything that we haven't already agreed we would try.'

Placing a hand in his lap and squeezing the erection he had concealed in his trousers, she put her mouth against his and made the kiss long and lingering.

The movie was slow to start, with copyright warnings in a variety of languages being followed by a menu that wasn't co-operating with John's attempts to use the remote.

Sonia only became aware of the delay in the movie's presentation when Richard cheered good naturedly. As soon as she glanced in their direction, Joseph said, 'I don't think Roger needs to watch this movie.'

They all chuckled with ribald amusement and Sonia moved her mouth away from Roger and drew her hand from his crotch. Settling herself back on the arm of the seat, she kept her legs slightly apart knowing the view she would present if any of the guests deigned to look in her direction. The image of Sharon Stone in *Basic Instinct* repeatedly played through her mind, although Sonia knew her posture was nowhere near as reserved.

On screen, the film began with a powerful sex scene where the blonde heroine was eagerly kneeling in front of two men and taking both their erections into her mouth. The actress's lips were glossed with saliva and pre-come as she hungrily devoured one shaft and then the other. By the time the opening scene was coming to its conclusion, and the actress had been used vaginally and anally and was preparing to have her face doused with semen, everyone in Sonia's lounge had fallen quiet and become absorbed in the film.

'It's good, isn't it?' Sonia ventured.

'Very good,' John agreed, shifting awkwardly in his seat. His expression was almost pained as he moved and his half-drained tin of lager remained firmly wedged in his lap.

The movie shifted to the next scene where the blonde actress was accompanied by a dark-skinned woman wearing tight Lycra.

'You must let me borrow this when I get back,' John told Sonia.

'Why do you want to borrow it?' she asked innocently.

'To watch it at home,' John replied.

'But you're watching it now,' Sonia pressed. She made her tone sound frustratingly naive and she could see his reaction was somewhere between amusement and irritation. 'What can you do at home with the DVD that you can't do here?' she asked.

'I can't wank off while I'm watching it here,' John spluttered.

Richard and Joseph chuckled while they blushed. John's honesty seemed to have removed some of the tension from the air and she watched everyone take a fresh sip from their drinks.

When the laughter at John's outburst had died down, Sonia studied him levelly and said, 'If you want to wank, no one's stopping you.'

All four men regarded her in silence. Feeling that something more needed to be said, Sonia added, 'I'm thinking of wanking off to this myself. I'm not stopping any of you guys from doing the same.'

Delighted by their attention, she passed her beer can to one side and raised the hem of her skirt. As the four men watched, she pressed a hand against the centre of her sex and then shivered.

'Normally, when I'm playing with myself, I like to tease my clit,' she explained later. 'But, because I knew I was putting on a show for these guys, I pushed two fingers straight inside.'

Arousal from all the preparations she had made paid dividends, as Sonia's fingers slipped easily inside her sex. The lips of her labia spread wide apart and she could feel her hand becoming greasy with the rush of wetness.

The DVD was forgotten as everyone watched Sonia's 'impromptu' performance. Moving to the coffee table, slipping her skirt off as she walked, she paused before sitting down and stared curiously at the three men on the settee. 'Am I the only one wanking off to this movie?'

With only the mildest reservations being expressed, her three guests unfastened the zips at their jeans. All of them were already erect and the atmosphere in the room shifted from tense to electric. Sonia took a moment to admire their different sizes and shapes before settling herself on the coffee table. She sat so they could watch her playing while she watched them.

They were close enough to touch her but, after Richard had raised a tentative hand against her leg, and Sonia had politely said, 'You don't need to touch me. Just touch yourself,' they were all respectful of her limits.

The DVD remained forgotten, although Sonia could hear it playing behind her. The grunts, squeals and groans of the porn film were intermingled with the slurp of deep penetrations and a cheesy backing track.

And Sonia watched the three men stroking themselves as she fingered her sex. Her orgasm was frustratingly close and she knew it could have been hers in an instant. Because she was theatrically teasing fingers between her labia, and allowing them to see every portion of her exposed sex, the release remained maddeningly out of her reach.

'Come and kiss me, Roger,' she demanded.

Her husband was with her in a second. Kneeling between her legs, placing his mouth against first one thigh and then the other, he had instantly understood that she did not want him to kiss her face. Moving his mouth higher, trembling with his own excitement, Roger finally rubbed his nose against her knuckles, urging Sonia to move her fingers away. She let him touch his nose to her sex, and almost came in that moment.

Watching John, Richard and Joseph – each holding a fist tight around their shafts and all of them stroking vigorously – she wondered if she dared to take things further this evening. She and Roger had always agreed that their limitations would never extend to sexual contact with anyone else. But, as the arousal grew stronger, Sonia fantasised about having one of the guests in her mouth while taking another between her legs.

Roger chose that moment to dart his tongue against her clitoris. Her orgasm was strong and instantaneous.

'I came so hard on his face,' Sonia said afterwards. 'It was the strongest climax I've ever enjoyed.'

Her cry sounded louder than any of the fake orgasms from the DVD and she could see it was an inducement to make Richard and Joseph stroke more quickly. John's hand moved lazily up and down his thick erection and his quick gaze flitted from her sex to her eyes. Sonia shivered at the idea of having another orgasm because she knew she was going to have that pleasure as she stared directly at John.

Encouraged by Sonia's response, Roger lapped more urgently at her sex. Their marriage had taught him how she best liked to be pleased and he teased her pussy using all the skills that came from their years of practice together. Not that Sonia needed much teasing.

Staring fixedly at John, only shifting her gaze occasionally to watch Richard and Joseph as they stroked themselves more furiously, she found herself battling against the prospect of each climax rather than simply wallowing in the pleasure. The boldness of what they were doing, and the knowledge she could take things so much further if she wanted, would have been enough to make her scream with satisfaction. The added joy of having Roger lick her pussy meant that her pleasure was enormous.

'Are you sure you don't want us to help you?' John asked coyly.

She shook her head.

It occurred to her that she could remove her top, flash her bare breasts at the trio and demand that two of them suck on her nipples. The idea of doing that was enough to make her buck her hips hard against Roger's nose. He continued to slurp greedily against her sex as she crested another wave of release.

Sonia also thought of having Roger screw her while the others watched, but she thought that could lead them to believe they were in with a chance of using her in the same way, and she didn't want to falsely raise their hopes. Knowing that she and her husband would be able to make love once their guests had gone, Sonia blinked perspiration from her eyes and stared at John, Richard and Joseph. 'I just want to watch you all come,' she explained.

'Not a problem,' John replied. His hand began to work more quickly in his lap.

Following suit, and no longer making any pretence of watching the DVD, Richard and Joseph also began to stroke themselves with fresh urgency.

Roger took his wife to the point of another orgasm and, as she held herself on the point of release, Sonia grunted and cursed as she demanded one of them should come while she watched.

Richard and Joseph obliged. Pushing themselves from the settee and falling to their knees in front of the coffee table, they each stroked with renewed vigour. Sonia was in a haze of bliss as she watched and enjoyed her husband's tongue against her sex. But that pleasure grew stronger when Richard reached his climax and spurted a string of semen across her carpet. She fought against the pull of orgasm long enough to watch Joseph's erection erupt and then demanded that John had to come now, while she watched.

Richard and Joseph moved out of John's way as he knelt on the floor and Sonia got her first proper look at their friend's cock. Because so many of hers and Roger's un-realised fantasies had involved John the nearness of his exposed erection was almost enough to make her climax on the spot. Taking in every detail of size, colour and contours, she watched his hand slide briskly back and forth as he pulled himself quickly to the point of release.

Roger's head remained buried between her legs. The waves of pleasure built quickly to a point where she could no longer fight them. And John stared into her eyes as his erection spat a load of white semen across the lounge carpet. Sonia roared as she savoured the strongest orgasm of the night.

* * *

'We've done similar things since then but it's always been soft swinging,' Sonia explained. 'And I think it always will be. When John came back from Germany, he'd brought a couple of new DVDs and we watched them together. It was a lot of fun. But John knew I didn't want him to touch me. Only watch. I get excited – I get *very* excited – by the thought of doing more with another man. But I know I would feel wrong about it afterwards. Having three men watch my husband eat my pussy was incredible. Seeing them tug off while they watched really did give me the strongest orgasm ever. But I know, if I did more than that, I would feel as though I was being unfaithful. And that's something I could never do.'

Xia

'the gang-bang girl'

'I've got the most bizarre story for you.'

Xia is 29 years old and considers herself a veteran of the swinging scene. Attractive, petite with jet-black hair and obvious oriental heritage in her features, she talks quickly and confidently. During our interview, she is dressed in a pair of designer jeans, comfortable trainers and a baggy pink sweatshirt that disguises her slender body and is emblazoned with the FCUK logo. Smoking coolly on a Marlboro Light, she admits that she has been sexually active since the age of fourteen and, before the age of seventeen, she had experienced her first threesome.

'After that, I didn't want to go back,' Xia confesses. 'It was important to me that every boyfriend I had should be into sharing and group stuff or I just sacked him off. I have a very high sex drive. When people ask me my favourite sexual position, I'm honest and say that I love being sandwiched between two well-hung guys. I don't like being unfaithful to guys, especially when we're meant to be boyfriend and girlfriend, but I'll screw behind their backs if they try to put restraints on my behaviour. My current guy has a couple of obliging friends who regularly call round on us so we can all enjoy ourselves together.'

She shakes her head, squashes her cigarette on the ashtray on my desk and reminds me that we were going to talk about the night she went to a party and became 'the gang-bang girl'.

I set the tape recorder, grab a paper and pen, and prepare to take notes. The tape recorder is a necessity because, although Xia paints a detailed picture of what happens, she speaks so quickly it's difficult to follow her story.

'It was the strangest evening of my life,' Xia begins.

Xia drew a deep breath before entering the house. She had received the address from a friend of a friend who knew she was a swinger. Details of the party – several couples and a handful of select singles gathering at a private house in Bristol – were scant, but sufficient to catch Xia's interest. Between partners, and deciding she needed the thrill of some self-affirming casual sex, Xia had decided she owed herself a night away from the misery of loneliness and something to distract her from the ennui of her position as PA to an executive in a large insurance company. A tingle of apprehension bristled through her but, brushing that aside, she knocked loudly on the door and waited for someone to answer.

'I'd been to these events before and this was a full-on thing where everything seemed to be happening. The majority of the people there were couples, but I saw quite a few singles too. Whoever had hosted the event had brought the right people together because, even though I only arrived half an hour late, things were already going hard when I showed up.'

Xia walked down a long hallway and into a large, dimly lit room. The smell of cigarettes mingled with the more distinctive zest of marijuana, thickening the air to an unbreathable smoke. Before she had entered the lounge, she was already feeling overdressed in her mini-skirt, stockings and long-line jacket. Previous experience at swingers' parties had taught her that participants were difficult to shock and she was exhibitionistic enough to want to make an impact. Consequently, Xia had elected to wear as little as possible and hoped to be seen as daring by those she met this evening. However, because she had arrived half an hour late, she could see that no one was going to be impressed by her state of undress when so many of the party's participants were already naked.

'No one seemed to be wearing clothes except me. Couples were fucking in the hallway as I was led through to the lounge. Some of them were walking around naked and not caring about it. A few of them were running around, chasing after each other, giggling and laughing. As I entered the lounge, I saw one woman being spit-roasted by two guys. She had a guy in her pussy and another one deep in her mouth. There were two really sexy-looking girls sucking face and fingering each other. Their boyfriends, husbands or whatever the fuck they were were standing over them and watching with really avid interest.

'It all seemed pretty much like a normal swingers' party, until the host – Frank I think his name was – pointed at me and shouted, "Here she is. Here she is!"'

The cry confused Xia and made her more than a little nervous. She freely admits that she was usually apprehensive when attending a swingers' party, and that anxiety was always heightened if she ever went alone. But, on every other previous occasion, the hosts and guests had gone out of their way to make her feel welcome and accepted.

'Usually, I can find someone to hook up with,' she explains. 'And, by the nature of the parties, if you're there with one person, you're there with all of them. But this cry singled me out. It made me feel uncomfortable and scared and I could have happily turned around and fled right then.'

Heads turned. Intimacies were forgotten as couples glanced in Xia's direction and then turned to look expectantly at Frank. Expectations were clearly raised and, to Xia's mounting horror, she heard someone echo Frank's cry and alert the rest of the house.

'She's here! Frank says she's here!'

Frank stepped to Xia's side and introduced himself. Although his exclamation had unsettled her, he was disarmingly pleasant. Naked, a decent-sized length dangling innocuously between his legs, he kissed her on each cheek before wrapping an arm around her waist. Xia noticed his penis began to grow stiffer as he pressed himself close.

'Here she is,' Frank called again. 'Here's our gang-bang girl.'

Xia swallowed and stared at him in amazement.

Frank briefly explained, because she had been the last one to arrive, she'd won the honour of becoming the evening's gang-bang girl. Not sure she understood what he was talking about, Xia pressed him for an explanation. 'What's a gang-bang girl?'

He laughed. 'A gang-bang girl is the girl who we're all going to gang-bang.'

If the words had been said to any other woman at any other party, Xia knows they would have inspired terror. With disarming honesty she confesses that, because she was alone, and had yet to encounter anyone she recognised from previous parties, she was feeling more than a little unnerved by Frank having awarded her such an unusual spot prize. Yet she was also excited.

'I'd been horny as I prepared for the party. I was suffering the usual nervous bouts, wondering if I was going to end up with anyone and whether or not it would be satisfying, or at least different enough to justify my involvement with swinging. What Frank was offering was something I'd never had before and I was eager to give it a try.'

'OK,' Xia told him. 'I'm tonight's gang-bang girl.' She smiled easily around the room and saw nods of approval and glances of raw and lusty appreciation.

'OK,' Frank repeated. He continued to hold Xia's hand high in the air. In a heavy and affected accent he shouted, *The gang-bang girl says yes.*

The words received a cheer.

Someone passed Xia a drink, as Frank led her to the large settee in the centre of the room. The words 'gang-bang girl' were shouted around the house and, while she wasn't particularly listening for the sound, Xia became aware of dozens of footsteps growing heavier as though people were rushing to see her. Her stomach folded with disquiet and, although she was still looking forward to being the gang-bang girl, she began to wonder if she had agreed to more than she was truly willing to give.

Men and women began to appear in the room, surprising her with their large numbers. She could see between fifteen and twenty couples as well as roughly the same amount of singles. The majority were naked; some continued to touch and maintain an intimacy, but it seemed as though everyone in the party had come to take a cursory glance at the gang-bang girl.

'From what I heard afterwards,' Xia explains, 'the party had started early. I don't know if it's just one of those rumours that gets spread around, but I'd been told that the first guests to arrive had been treated to the sight of the host and hostess "playing" with their dog. I don't know if there was any truth in the story, or if it was just said to add to the atmosphere of "we will fuck anything", but, apparently, she was on her knees, sucking her husband's dick, while the dog straddled her from behind.' Conspiratorially, Xia adds, 'I did see a dog mooching around the house later on – it was a Great Dane, lying in a basket in the kitchen – but that doesn't mean a lot. Plenty of these stories get bandied around at parties and they get exaggerated to ridiculous points. The only problem with a swingers' party is that you have to go to some pretty excessive lengths to exaggerate the events. I mean, who would believe I could go to a party, get fucked thirty times and still stagger out of the party craving another cock?' She laughs, shakes her head and adds, 'It crossed my mind to wonder, if the host was getting the dog to help spit-roast his wife when the first couple arrived, who opened the door for them?' She raises an eyebrow as though proving a point. Wafting smoke aside from a second Marlboro Light, she adds, 'But I never asked because that would have been rude and you simply don't call people bullshit artists at swingers' parties. That sort of behaviour can really spoil the atmosphere.'

A couple of women joined Frank and helped Xia to get comfortable. One of them was naked, her large breasts brushing against Xia each time she pressed closer. The other wore black lace panties, stockings and a matching bra. The lingerie looked new and exotic and made Xia wish she had worn something equally feminine and flattering. Eagerly, both women kissed and touched her. Although Xia responded to them both, she admits that the party was not like anything she had been to before.

'I don't know if Frank had picked on me because, with me having an oriental look, I was something new and different. Or if he had previously decided that the last woman in would be the gang-bang girl. Or if this was something he did at all his parties. All I knew was that I was the centre of attention in a room full of naked and semi-naked strangers and two beautiful women were kissing me and trying to turn me on. I'd barely had a chance to take a swig at my tin of lager. It really was like nothing I'd ever experienced before.'

Xia felt a hand slip inside her jacket. Warm, feminine fingers cupped one breast and stroked her rigid nipple. Xia's head was held tight, her face fixed in position so the woman in the black lingerie could extract a long lingering kiss. Her tongue glided easily into Xia's mouth. The taste of something sweet and darkly alcoholic flavoured the exchange. A flush of air touched Xia's stomach as her jacket was opened, exposing her bare stomach to the room. She was distantly aware of a ripple of approval travelling through those guests watching.

'If the two women thought they were getting me warmed up with foreplay, they were seriously mistaken. I'd walked into the room nervous but, as soon as Frank called me the gang-bang girl, my arousal had kicked in. When they started kissing me, I was into them the same way I'd be into a woman an hour after we'd started to touch. My nipples were hard, my pussy was wet and repeatedly clenching and I was desperate for physical contact. To me, those kisses weren't foreplay. They were my first sex of the evening.'

Xia's jacket was eased from her shoulders. Because she only wore a mini and stockings underneath, the removal left her nearly naked. A loud murmur of approval went through the crowd this time but Xia barely heard the sound. Engrossed in being caressed by one woman while kissing another, she allowed them to unfasten her skirt and expose the secrets of her cleanly shaven sex.

The naked woman pulled Xia's face away from her friend and demanded her own kiss. The woman in the black pants, bra and stockings took advantage of the moment and pressed her warm mouth over Xia's breast. Her body was sandwiched between expanses of soft bare flesh; the smell of semen, sex juices and sweat permeated the air; the atmosphere of arousal, throbbing through the party, made her weak with need.

'And I'd been there less than five minutes.'

She was guided to the settee and admits that, if she hadn't been helped to sit down, she would have collapsed. Her shoulders were pushed back into the welcoming leather as the two women joined her. Thoroughly involved with the pair, Xia remained oblivious to the rest of the room. Even when strange hands clutched at her stocking-clad ankles, she didn't bother to glance at whoever was touching her. Engrossed in the act of being kissed and fondled, she allowed her legs to be stroked, caressed and then pulled wide apart.

It was only when she felt an erection probe the lips of her sex that Xia remembered she was genuinely going to be the gang-bang girl.

'The idea thrilled me,' she admits. 'One of the women had been calling me a lucky bitch, but I thought she was just jealous because I'm stunning and good looking. It was only when I felt that first cock sliding inside me that I realised I'd won a prize that nearly every other woman in the room had wanted.'

Her pussy was wet and ready for him. He slipped inside so easily she could see he was truly surprised by the speed with which penetration occurred. His eyes opened wide, as his smile grew broader, and then he was pushing in deeper and with more urgency.

The pungent scent of her sex was stronger than she had expected. The thrill of being ridden by this stranger, while the two unknown women continued to kiss and fondle, made for a potent aphrodisiac. Breathless with arousal, and eagerly responding to stimulation, Xia could feel her body rushing towards the first orgasm of the evening.

'I don't know if the group had planned out how they were going to use 'the gang-bang girl' when she arrived. The women were at my top half, kissing my mouth, sucking my nipples, stroking me and touching my breasts. On those few occasions when I pulled my face away from the women above me, I could see the guys were forming a queue. It truly was like nothing I have ever experienced before. I've had two or three guys in one evening. The night I had four guys I managed to slip two of them into my pussy at the same time while I sucked the other two off. But even that experience, as good as it was, was nothing like this. *I have never felt so turned on.*'

Laughing, she admits, 'It crossed my mind that my behaviour would be seen as slutty if anyone ever discovered what I had done. But that would only have been the attitude I would have got from those who don't swing. Within the crowd at the party, I knew I was envied by the women and wanted by the men. One of the girls kissing me called me a lucky bitch again and, as the first guy grunted and then climaxed inside me, I agreed with her.'

Xia was in no mood to count heads or gather too many details about the events of the gang-bang. She knows there were more than twenty men at the party but believes only fifteen or so had turned up to enjoy her gang-bang. Constantly kissing and being kissed; savouring the sensation of having a stranger's erection slide into her; enjoying the thrill of being ridden by someone she didn't know; then delighting in the sensation of that man's spent cock being replaced by a fresh one; Xia had lost interest in the world beyond her own body and its responses.

Her shoes were removed and one of her stockings was peeled from her thigh. Xia was treated to the disquieting sensation of having her toe sucked. She didn't know if the mouth at her foot belonged to a man or a woman and, because the sensation wasn't totally unpleasant, she allowed it to continue as another erection slipped between her swollen sex lips and another woman stole a kiss from her mouth.

'There were fifteen or more guys in the lounge,' she said afterwards. 'And I'm pretty sure each one of them had me at least twice. For the best part of two hours I was sprawled on the settee, being kissed and suckled by horny women while man after man fucked me. It was truly intense. My pussy grew sore early on in the evening but the burning sensation only added to the pleasure.' She snorts laughter, stretches her smile to a wicked grin and adds, 'Admittedly, in the week after, I came down with the nastiest case of thrush I've ever suffered. But that was an after-effect and it didn't spoil the night itself. I suppose, if that burning sensation was a warning of what was going to come, I could enjoy suffering that sort of warning a lot more often.'

All the men wore condoms. The clinical scent of lubricated prophylactics carried over the fragrances of perspiration, spunk and feminine musk.

Yet Xia still believed the evening was the most bizarre she had ever enjoyed. 'The strange thing was, although I was really enjoying being the centre of attention: I wanted more. I had all these beautiful women kissing me, and more men than I was sure I could handle: but I wanted more. I wanted to suck on a guy's cock and I wanted to swallow his come.'

She murmured the request to one of the women kissing her. An excess of pleasure had already slurred her speech and made her inarticulate but Xia believes she expressed herself clearly enough. 'I want to suck cock.'

'You've got enough cock,' the woman growled. Grabbing Xia's hair and pulling so their faces met, she whispered, 'Put this in your mouth, instead.'

The kiss silenced Xia's pleas to satisfy her craving. And, as another stranger rode her to the point of a brutal, satisfying orgasm, she tried to convince herself that her body did not need to suck a cock for that final rush of pleasure.

'I don't count orgasms,' she said afterwards. 'So I can't tell you how many times I came. But I do know I came often and I came very hard. Every now and again I'd find myself being ridden by someone who knew what they were doing and the climax would build inside me. It would only take the kiss of one of the women, or the touch of a hand against my breast, and then I'd be screaming with pleasure. My pussy muscles would go into a furious spasm and I'd be groaning and thrashing and nearly crippled with the strength of each orgasm. I'm surprised I didn't piss myself with the force of some of the orgasms,' she adds honestly. 'Every moment I was there was all about my pleasure. The women kissing and sucking me were taking me to a real high. My pussy was being filled and used by so many decent cocks I could barely think straight. I've never enjoyed such intense and satisfying pleasure. But I craved that one more thing.'

'I want to suck a cock,' Xia gasped. The cry came out sounding pitiful and pathetic. It was an hour into the gang-bang and the hammering between her legs had been relentless. She didn't know if the women kissing her were the same ones she had encountered at the start of the evening or if they had changed as her face was pulled from one to the other. All she knew was that she had to make her needs known to someone. 'I want to suck cock and I want to swallow a good dollop of wet salty come.'

'You filthy bitch.' The blonde kissing her giggled. Clearly excited by the suggestion, the blonde kissed more ferociously.

Xia immediately understood she was not going to get the response she wanted. Torn by unparalleled feelings of frustration and satisfaction, she groaned with despair as another orgasm trembled through the inner muscles of her sex.

'Please,' she begged. The words came out in an articulate wail of tears. 'Please. Someone. Let me suck your cock.' Her cries were stifled as a woman placed her mouth over Xia's and tongue-wrestled her to silence.

Another erection replaced the spent one inside her pussy and then a fresh stiffness was pounding and pounding inside the burning muscles of her sex.

'I always try and practise safe sex when I'm at a party,' Xia explains. 'But it's never as easy as the experts make it sound. You make a decision before you leave that you're not going to do anything without a condom but it doesn't always happen that way. Sometimes, when you're really horny, the idea of waiting for a guy to search around for his pants and find his packet of condoms is too much of a delay. By the time he's got himself some protection the idea of screwing him has passed, or you're fucking his best friend instead.' She sniggers, as though the comment reminds her of something funny. With the laughter still in her voice, she says, 'It's far simpler, although probably not quite as wise, to think, "Fuck waiting", and then do the guy there and then. I know people are all into safe sex these days but, speaking for my own preferences, I do love the feel of a bare cock inside my pussy.'

Expounding on the topic of condoms, Xia adds, 'I should say, when you make a decision that you're not going to do anything without a condom, that doesn't apply to blowjobs where I'm concerned. The damned things taste so fucking awful I can't imagine why anyone would want one in their mouth. Oral sex is supposed to be a really sensuous experience; you're supposed to be tasting the guy's cock: not just rubbing your tongue against him; and I'm sure I've read that there's virtually no chance of the more serious diseases being passed on by blowjobs. So I never use them for oral.' She sneers with disgust, lights a fresh cigarette and adds, 'Even when they're supposedly flavoured with mint or fruit or chocolate, they still taste of condom or spermicide. I guess they can make them taste so lousy because no woman is going to send a letter to them and say, "I was sucking my boyfriend the other night while he wore one of your fruit-flavoured condoms and I have to say the flavour was absolutely sickening. Please refund my money and make it publicly known that I am a disgruntled customer."' She giggles at the idea, wafts her cigarette across the room again, and continues to relate the details of her bizarre evening as the gang-bang girl.

Bathed in sweat, cresting on a level of pleasure that went beyond anything she had ever experienced during a regular relationship, Xia accepted the kisses of the women and continued to bask in the pleasure of having repeated men thrust between her legs. She occasionally glanced at the strangers as they took her. Their sizes, lengths, thickness and techniques had become indistinguishable. The barrage of pleasure was relentless and Xia gave herself to the experience without reservation.

One thoughtful woman handed her a glass of beer. She had managed to sip at her first but it had been lost during the two hours she had been trapped on the settee under a constant stream of men. Now she drank this one, quenching a thirst she had barely noticed and wishing she was drinking something warmer and more viscous. As she sipped the cool lager from the glass, another man ejaculated inside her and then another took his place between her legs.

Some of the icy liquid spilled against her bare breasts, causing her to flinch as she realised how hot her body had become. A redhead licked the amber fluid away, smiling up at Xia as her tongue stroked daringly close to one stiff nipple. Her green eyes shone mischievously and her darkly painted lips encircled the hard bead of flesh.

Xia stiffened as another orgasm battered its way through her aching body.

And the men continued to take her. Their stamina seemed to have improved and, rather than a few thrusts and a squirt, she was now being pounded long and hard by each new man who straddled himself between her spread thighs. Absently, she noticed that her other stocking had gone. She realised her foot was wet and wondered if the toe-sucker had been at her without her realising. The idea didn't unsettle her – she had been enjoying a sensory overload throughout the evening and she didn't doubt the toe-sucker contributed in some small way to her excess of pleasure.

She knew that some of the men had entered her, climaxed and been replaced without her breaking her kiss from one of the women at her face, so the thought of someone sucking at her toe without her knowledge was barely worthy of concern. But she did wonder where her stockings had gone.

And she still craved the taste of having an erection ejaculate in her mouth.

'By the end of the experience, I'd just about had enough,' Xia admits. 'Considering the thrush that hit me afterwards, I think I'd had more than enough. Maybe too much. But I still wanted to taste some cock. I told the blonde girl who'd been sucking my nipples while I was gang-banged. I said I was desperate to taste a cock.'

'You're a greedy bitch, aren't you?' the blonde gasped. 'Haven't you had enough cock?'

'I've had plenty of cock,' Xia agreed. 'But I didn't get to taste any.'

The last man pulled away from her with a breathless thank you. Xia saw his length was now flaccid and his condom was made heavy from his spend. Her own juices stained the side of the prophylactic and her stomach felt heavy with disdain as she realised she had missed another chance to satisfy her craving.

The blonde frowned as she noticed Xia's upset, her expression of disdain implying that Xia was some sort of cock-hungry ingrate who couldn't even be satisfied by a dozen or more swingers screwing her twice.

'I tried to point out that I'd had more than enough cock between my legs but I was still anxious to taste come. Yet I don't think it sank in. She said she'd go and find her husband, or some guy who was up for being swallowed, and then she got me another beer and I was left alone on the settee.'

Xia remained alone on the settee for a further half an hour before the need to pee urged her to move. With urination, she suffered terrible kidney pains, which she said she had never had before, or since.

After leaving the bathroom, she staggered naked around the house, watching other couples, triples and foursomes fucking, before realising she was alone and unwanted at the party. After visiting the kitchen to get herself a fresh beer, walking gingerly past the intimidating bulk of the Great Dane, she went back to the settee in the hope of finding enough of her clothes to make her return home.

'There were still other couples all around me. But it's always been my experience at parties that the sex comes in a mad rush either at the beginning, middle or end. The rest of the time is either spent in a haze of expectation, anticipation or disappointment. This one seemed to be the exception because, even though all the guys had been through me, they were still up for having as much fun as they could. I don't know if the hosts had invited this specific group of guests because of the men's stamina, or if the women in the group were just adamant that they were going to have their fun before they went home. Whatever the reason for everyone's excessive appetites, I sat alone – sipping my beer and wanting to taste come – and knowing it wasn't going to happen there. No one spoke to me as I slipped on my jacket, retrieved my skirt and then hobbled to the door.' With a tight-lipped smile she adds, 'I never did find my stockings.'

Leaning forwards in her seat, remaining serious as she nears the end of her narrative, Xia says, 'I took a taxi home. I was living alone at the time, and I sat in the back feeling miserable and peculiarly unsatisfied. The taxi driver asked me if I'd been to a party, and if I was OK. Chancing a desperate gambit, I said I was OK, but I'd feel better if I could suck a guy's cock. Predictably enough, he volunteered and I got him to pull over at the side of the road. He came in the back of the cab with me, rather than trusting me in the front, but that didn't trouble me at all. I was just happy to have my lips around a length of meat. And I don't know why I was so hungry for the taste of it that evening. I don't know if all the fucking had made me desperate for the flavour, or if it was just one of those impulse things you get that leave you needing a particular taste in your mouth. Whatever the reason, I went down on him, licked him hard and then sucked him dry. His cock wasn't particularly big or thick or good in any way. But the flavour of his semen was exactly what I needed. When he jetted at the back of my throat, I actually came, and it was the orgasm I remember as being the best of the evening.'

Sitting back, she adds, 'Didn't I tell you it was a bizarre story? I got to be the gang-bang girl at a swingers' party. I got screwed by two dozen guys and, in total, I must have been fucked thirty or forty times. I had the most beautiful women kissing me, sucking my tits and some weirdo licking my toes. And my best orgasm came from sucking off a cabbie in exchange for the ride home.'

Larry & Cora
'R U UP 4 IT?'

L arry excuses himself and goes to the bathroom, leaving Cora alone with the two strangers. The need to pee is not at the forefront of his mind. But, once alone, he reaches for something small from the front of his jeans pocket and fumbles with it for a short while.

Then he presses the button to send the text message.

'R U UP 4 IT?'

'I don't know how people used to swing before the invention of mobile phones,' Larry confides. 'When you're face to face with another couple, it's impossible to ask your partner, "Do you want to screw either of these two?" without causing offence. Discreet whispers look rude. Code words are too obvious. But a simple question in a text message, and a yes or no response, has always worked for me and Cora. I truly envy these couples who can read each other's mind. I always have a fair idea of what Cora wants but I like to get a firm commitment before I go ahead and put us in a situation that might prove embarrassing if I've misread the signs. If she sends back a message that says "NO", or "NOT SURE", I would never push it.'

His mobile emits two short beeps to announce the receipt of a response. The screen glows for an instant before he glances at it, smiles and then pockets the phone.

The message said simply: O YES.

After flushing the lavatory and quickly washing his hands, Larry makes his way down the stairs to find his wife and their new friends. The house is one of the new-build properties that he and Cora have often argued over. He considers them to be too small, poorly built (he is in the construction industry and privy to the worst secrets of the new housing industry) but he knows Cora likes their unsullied newness. This one is still new enough to be fragranced with the scents of wet paint and Larry grudgingly concedes that it is an attractive property, although he still believes it is too compact for his tastes. The lavatory is at the top of the short flight of stairs and, by the time he has reached the bottom, he is in their hosts' lounge where Cora and Anita are kissing.

Damien, Anita's husband, watches with lascivious interest. Larry can find no reason to condemn Damien's expression because he knows his own appraisal is little short of a leer. Making himself comfortable in a seat facing them, he grins and says, 'I see you ladies have started without me.'

The kiss is a splendid display of exhibitionism. Cora has her hand against the side of Anita's head, her fingers resting lightly beneath a fringe of blonde curls and touching one bronzed cheek. Anita has her fingertips touching Cora's throat. Because Anita is a suntanned blonde and Cora is a monochrome Goth, the pair look like a meeting of alien cultures. Both women have recently applied lipstick, making their mouths ripe and succulent. They taste each other, tongues slipping against teeth and brushing over lips before gliding together. Their eyes are initially guarded; they wear hesitant expressions, but then they smile as the thrill of what they are doing takes over.

Cora finally breaks the kiss and glances over at Larry. Her wan skin is made paler by the accent of dark eye shadow and hair that is oil-slick black. The lilt of her regional brogue adds a seductive charm to every word she mutters. 'Of course we started without you.' She laughs. 'Me and Anita don't need you for this, now, do we?'

She makes the statement as she shrugs off her jacket. The top she wears is sheer and lacy. It had looked like a delicate blouse while covered by the lapels but, now that it can be seen in its entirety, it is revealed as a filmy gauze of sheer fabric that clings revealingly to the bare flesh of her shoulders, sides and breasts. The dark circles of her areolae are visible through the flimsy net and everyone in the room can see her stiff nipples.

Cora blushes lightly when she realises they are all staring. Even though the smiles are appreciative, and this was close to the effect she had yearned for when she selected the body-stocking, the attention is sufficient to make her cheeks turn a very un-Gothlike shade of pink.

'You came all the way down here wearing that?' Anita gasps. Her tone is a mixture of amazement and amusement.

Cora shrugs as though her boldness is of little consequence. 'I wanted to look good for the two of you.'

'You managed that well enough,' Damien comments.

Cora stretches her smile to include him but her gaze remains fixed on Anita. 'Do you like?' she asks. Glancing down at herself, idly stroking the bud of one nipple, she raises a questioning eyebrow and asks, 'It's not too daring, is it? It doesn't make me look cheap or slutty, do you think?'

The see-through blouse is a transparent body-stocking, decorated so it looks like it has been spun from spider-webs. It is very much in keeping with Cora's vampish image and, although the black net makes her skin look grey, the garment can only be described as flattering.

There is a moment's silence as Anita and Damien consider how to reply. Before Damien can speak, Anita lunges forwards and kisses Cora again. This time there is a hearty enthusiasm in the exchange where there was previously nervousness. As the blonde crushes her lips against Cora's, her hands begin to explore. Cora's breasts are caressed through the thin film of fabric that covers them. The nipples grow more rigid and both women are soon breathless with rising arousal.

'Is this what you expected it would be?' Larry asks Damien.

Neither woman bothers to look at him. They are too involved in the discovery of kissing each other.

Damien shifts awkwardly in his seat, clearly aroused but obviously embarrassed. Despite Larry's affable smile, and the fact that this is his home, he seems to be having difficulty feeling at ease. 'I didn't think . . .' He stops, shakes his head and smiles before starting again. 'I didn't think we'd ever have the courage to go through with this,' he manages.

Damien is as pale in skin tone as Cora, bespectacled and has his blond hair cropped short, neat and tidy. Although he is wearing jeans and a T-shirt he looks like an off-duty office worker and it is easy to imagine him in a shirt and tie.

'And is it what you expected?' Larry presses. 'Is this how you imagined your Anita would look while she's kissing another woman?'

Damien watches Cora and Anita for a moment longer before responding.

Anita's blouse is open. Cora has a hand inside and whatever it is her fingers are doing the movement is exciting both women. Anita continues to touch Cora's thinly veiled breasts while their mouths join in a slippery union of passion. Together they are panting and hungrily pressing into each other.

'I never thought we'd get to do this,' Damien says eventually.

Cora pulls her face from Anita's lips and looks kindly at him. 'You'll both get to do a lot more before the night's over.' She glances slyly at Larry and then adds, 'At least, you will if you're up for it.'

Partly to show off for their men, but mainly because this is what Anita and Cora have been eagerly anticipating, the two women begin to undress as they experiment with each other. This is Anita's first time with another woman and she is initially hesitant about touching Cora. Her reservations are short-lived and she is soon sucking on one nipple through the flimsy garment while Cora carefully peels away her blouse, her skirt and then her underwear. It takes a while before Anita is naked but, because she is lost in the thrill of being intimate with Cora, she has no reservations about losing her clothes. Her breasts are plump, firm and marked with white triangles where her bikini has modestly covered her. As the rest of her body is exposed she reveals a pale triangle of flesh over her crotch.

Her sex is bereft of hair and Larry is in the perfect position to see that her labia are small and thin, neatly contained in the slit of her sex. He is able to watch his wife's fingers part the pussy lips and slide easily inside. The erection he has been sporting for the last half-hour aches for release.

As her fingers glide in and out of Anita's sex, Cora lowers herself down the woman's body and begins to lap gently against the musky wetness. Her smile is wary – as though she is half expecting Anita to resist or suddenly refuse the attention – and so she keeps the kisses light at first until she has stirred enough excitement to make Anita want more.

'Why don't you kiss your wife while Cora's playing with her?' Larry suggests.

Damien nods eagerly but makes no move to join the two women on the settee.

Cora uses both hands to expose the bare flesh of Anita's pussy and places a lingering kiss against her wetness. Mesmerised, Damien watches for a moment longer before standing up and smiling down at his beloved Anita. The adoration in his eyes is matched by her expression of decadent happiness. And then the pair kiss furiously as Cora laps greedily at the blonde's sex.

'Are you enjoying yourself down there, my love?' Larry asks.

He kneels beside Cora, one hand resting easily on her backside. His fingers tease idly against the crotchless gusset of her body-stocking and he gently explores her sex. The flesh is sopping with arousal and he penetrates her without any effort.

Cora moans as she buries her tongue deep inside Anita. The blonde gasps and begins to urgently try and open Damien's jeans. Eager to participate, Damien struggles to unfasten the awkward buttons at his fly.

Within two minutes, the foursome are joined together: Damien's penis is in Anita's mouth; Anita's pussy is around Cora's tongue; and Cora's pussy is squeezing around Larry's erection.

Clothes are discarded haphazardly around the room, although Cora still wears her gothic body-stocking. Cora is the mother of two children (one to Larry and another from an earlier relationship) and she is self-conscious about her not-quite-flat stomach. Consequently, she takes every opportunity to conceal this feature when there is a chance it might be seen by another couple. And, when she murmurs words of appraisal about Anita's figure, the compliments are genuine and heartfelt. She truly appreciates the chance to enjoy a body as lovely as Anita's and she pays homage to it with every gentle kiss she delivers to her inner thighs, labia and clitoris.

Anita comes with an anguished scream. She has one hand on the top of Cora's head and the other clutches Damien's backside as she tries to encourage him to thrust further into her mouth. Her mood of obvious abandon is infectious and, as Larry chuckles, Cora vents her own sigh of elation.

The room is not particularly warm but everyone glistens with perspiration.

'Different position,' Larry decides. He draws the back of his hand across his brow, removing a veneer of sweat.

'Yes,' Anita agrees, gasping the word as though she is either thirsty or desperate for air. Glancing down at Cora, smiling determinedly, she says, 'I want to do that to you. I want to do it now.'

'You can both do it together,' Larry says. Moving Cora aside, he gallantly helps Anita from the settee and guides her to lie on a coffee table in the centre of the floor. Although they are both naked, and in states of extreme arousal, there is a surprising amount of propriety between the couple. Larry is careful not to touch Anita's breasts, sex or backside, and he makes no acknowledgement towards having observed her nudity or arousal. Her nipples stand erect. Her sex lips, which had been contained in a neat slit at her cleft, are now a flushed-pink pout that drips with wetness. His sheathed erection occasionally brushes Anita's thigh, as he makes sure she is comfortable, but neither of them appears to notice. The predefined arrangement was that only the two women would be swinging together on this occasion and neither Larry nor Anita wants to renege on this agreement.

'Cora, my love,' Larry calls. He extends a hand for his partner and she comes quickly to his side. Encouraging her to assume a 69 position with Anita, guiding Cora into the superior position with Anita underneath, he asks, 'Why don't you and Anita enjoy each other a little more while Damien and I watch?'

'Is that what you two would like?' Cora asks, glancing first at Anita then at Damien.

The couple don't bother to consult and nod eagerly.

And so both women fall together, faces pressed against pussies as they greedily lick, lap and nuzzle. The sound of their slurping fills the room. Larry watches with an appreciative smile; Damien stares on in bewilderment. The sultry perfume of sexual secretions flavours every breath, and the electric mood of excitement continues to grow stronger.

Anita climaxes for a second time, but her cries are muffled as she buries her face against the wet folds of Cora's sex. She complains that Cora is doing the cunnilingus too well – not giving her the opportunity to reciprocate – and

Cora asks if she'd prefer for Larry to do it, 'because he's crap with his tongue'.

They all chuckle at the joke but the mirth is banished as the two men join in. Larry slides his sheathed erection into Cora. Damien pushes himself into his wife. The mood of light-hearted fun disappears as the four suddenly become serious and earnest in their pursuit of pleasure. Anita and Cora continue to lick and lap at each other, their efforts made awkward by the erections that are now buried in the holes they were kissing and their focus distracted as their personal enjoyment begins to build.

Anita encourages both Damien and Cora with pleas for more. Larry clutches tightly at his wife's hips and pushes himself deeper inside. He is not surprised to feel Anita's tongue slip against his shaft as he penetrates his wife but he deliberately stops himself from thinking that Cora is probably treating Damien to the same sly pleasure.

From previous experience, he knows that she will confess that indiscretion to him later when they are enjoying the magnificent sex that always comes after an episode of swinging. She will kiss him, tell him that he's just tasted a tongue that was recently sliding against another man's cock, and his climax will come in a glorious and sudden release that satisfies them both.

But, for now, intent on making this moment last as long as possible and be enjoyable for all those involved, he brushes that impending conversation from his mind and fixes his thoughts on pleasing his wife.

The end comes in a satisfying rush for all of them. Damien explodes inside Anita and the force of his orgasm causes her to climax. He pushes himself into her with a violent shudder that goes unnoticed as Larry and Cora wallow in their shared orgasms.

After pulling themselves apart, sighing, groaning and marvelling at the experience, the two couples fall back to their regular partners for an embrace that reaffirms their true affections.

Damien makes sure Anita is comfortable on the settee, and then, ever the polite host, he asks his guests if they would like a drink. Considering he was embarrassed about the whole situation at the start of the evening, he now appears comfortable as he stands naked in front of comparative strangers and offers them refreshments. He is even the first one to suggest that Larry and Cora should call on them again, in the near future, so they can enjoy this experience again and possibly take things further.

Cora goes to the loo after saying she wants to 'freshen up'.

Anita and Damien, still naked, lounge together on the settee. They constantly touch, stroke and caress, Damien pressing kisses against the back of her neck and Anita clearly revelling in the attention.

Larry sits alone with a glass of mineral water in his hand, exchanging pleasantries with the couple and enjoying the post-coital ambience, when he hears his mobile give the familiar two beeps that indicate a text message has been received. Rummaging through the discarded clothes to find his jeans, he pulls out his phone and reads the message from Cora.

'R U UP 4 2NDS?'

WHO SWINGS?

WHO SWINGS?

Culturally, some form of swinging has occurred through-out every episode of recorded history. The voyeuristic ritual of Hierosgamos in ancient Mesopotamia involved the country's ruler having public sex with a high-ranking hierodule (priestess) while an enthusiastic populace watched attentively. Cleopatra's voracious appetites – 100 noblemen in one night – have been meticulously recorded from the times of the Roman Empire. Lucrezia Borgia orchestrated the infamous 'chestnut orgy' in the Vatican. Casanova detailed an extensive diary of conquests in his *Histoire de Ma Vie*. The Marquis de Sade seemed unable to separate his private life from his novels of sexual cruelty and misogynistic debauchery. The Chukchee of Siberia made wife-lending contracts and, until the advent of Christian missionaries in Greenland, Eskimo men were known to make similar arrangements for their spouses.

Polygamy is frequently referenced throughout the Bible (Abraham, Israel, King David and Solomon) and Mormons embraced the practice until the church's then president, Joseph F Smith, denounced plural marriages in his 'Second Manifesto' of 1904. Advocates of Judaism enjoyed poly-gamy until the eleventh century, and it is still permissible within some factions of Islam, most particularly those in West Africa, Saudi Arabia and the United Arab Emirates. Although multiple marriages are now forbidden under Indian law, Hinduism, the religion followed by 98 per cent of the country's population, does not explicitly prohibit polygamy.

In the 1960s, sex parties were used as the central diversionary issue in the Profumo affair, drawing the focus of media attention away from a compromise to British security. In more recent times, the 2003 Christmas edition of the *A&F Quarterly*, distributed by the American clothiers Abercrombie & Fitch, strongly advocated group sex until the efforts of protestors saw that particular issue of the clothing catalogue pulled from distribution.

Anthropologically, group sex has been recorded amongst the habits of animals as varied as dolphins, snails, tree frogs and the legendary bonobo chimpanzees.

In short, swinging isn't limited to any demograph, race, era, religion, geographical location, social strata or even species. The only honest answer to the question 'Who swings?' is the simple response: swingers.

Vincent & Wendy
'. . . theology and the taxman's penis . . .'

A smouldering summer sun rests low in the sky above a leafy suburb of Nottingham's exclusive Park area. The smoky tang of the barbecue still perfumes the secluded garden and the scent makes the memory of the barbecue more appetising than the food had truly been. From somewhere inside the patio windows, a Norah Jones CD keeps the mood relaxed, informal and intimate.

The party has mellowed into polite groups who chat easily together. They stand outside, clustered together, sipping from their wineglasses and showing no hurry to end the day's sultry ambience.

Wendy has the largest group gathered before her and her cultured accent, matronly with round vowels, rings clearly through the air. She smiles with devilish humour and proclaims, 'Civil servants have the tiniest cocks.'

It is a bold statement and meets with admonishment from her husband of eleven years, Vincent. 'Not all civil servants have tiny cocks,' he corrects her. He flashes an embarrassed smile at the couple to whom the remark was principally directed.

Clearly flustered, they are both blushing. Newcomers to the swinging scene, the couple had solicited Wendy's opinion as to what happened at parties and what they should expect. The question 'Who swings?' had not been specifically raised, but their request for information was something similar.

Never afraid to offer a forthright rejoinder, Wendy is determined to make her point and she scowls at Vincent for his interruption.

'That's a gross generalisation,' Vincent tells her.

Wendy shrugs, confident in her facts and unwilling to recant the statement. 'It's true. All civil servants have tiny cocks. They get smaller depending on the department in which the civil servant works.'

Vincent rolls his eyes.

'Those who work in the pension's department probably have the biggest cocks,' Wendy concedes. 'But even those are small in comparison with the national average. The civil servants who work in the tax office have the smallest cocks.'

'Wendy!'

'Except for the women.'

Vincent studies his wife guardedly.

'The women don't have small cocks,' Wendy assures him. He looks ready to accept her contrite tone when Wendy trumpets, 'They have the fattest arses. And they have so much cellulite their buttocks look like the imitation leather sofas you sometimes see in the back alleys outside charity shops.'

Wendy's audience laughs indulgently. The only pair not laughing are the newbies who had earlier told Vincent that they work in the tax office. Blushes of fury, embarrassment and indignation now colour their previously pale cheeks. Their polite smiles look as brittle as shards of ice.

Ignoring her husband's attempts to be tactful, Wendy continues to extol the lack of virtues in having any member of the tax office present at a swingers' party.

Tall, blonde this week, and attractive in a lofty and superior fashion, Wendy works hard at a private gym to maintain a physique that looks like it belongs to a woman ten years her junior. She is dressed in clothes that are from the most stylish range of M&S and she strives for an image that is played down and unpretentious. 'I don't know why you're disagreeing with me, darling,' she admonishes Vincent. 'I thought we'd already agreed that tiny dicks and cellulite were God's punishment to people for choosing to work in the tax office?'

It's difficult to judge whether Wendy's generalisation comes from honest perception or a grudge against certain branches of the civil service. Quite possibly, it is a combination of the two because, whenever Wendy is questioned on a point, she backs it up with a strong argument.

'I don't think our guests want to hear about your opinions on theology and the taxman's penis,' Vincent complains.

Wendy is quick to respond. 'What was Fat Tony's cock like?'

'I don't know. I didn't see Fat Tony's cock. I was with Fat Tony's wife.'

'And did she have a cellulite problem?'

'She had cellulite. I don't know if she considered it a problem.'

'And did they both work in the tax office?'

'Just because those two worked in –'

'Did they both work in the tax office?'

Arguments at swingers' parties are not common. Experienced couples usually put disagreements aside until after the event, or find somewhere private to discuss anything more pressing. Newcomers, squabbling because of nervousness or reservations, will invariably leave the party or be encouraged to take their discussion somewhere less public.

Very experienced, Vincent and Wendy are not an exception to this rule. They both calm down the instant they realise their disagreement is making others uncomfortable. Staunching the difference of opinion before it can cause further angst, they kiss each other with mumbled apologies and make their peace.

As they embrace, Vincent whispers to his wife, 'Didn't you know? The newbies work in the tax office.'

Smiling with a look of pure mischief, Wendy replies, 'Yes, I know.'

Giggles from beside the barbecue draw everyone's attention. A summery blonde is treated to gentle applause now that she has removed her top. A long skirt still covers her waist, hips and legs, but the upper half of her sun-kissed body is exposed to the garden. She has full breasts. Her areolae are large, round and pale pink, and her nipples are already stiff. The gentleman to her left tentatively places his hand against one breast and gently strokes her. The lady on her right mirrors his actions.

'Damn.' Wendy frowns. 'I was hoping I'd be the first one to get my tits out this evening.'

'Perhaps you should consider keeping your mouth closed and your blouse open at the next party,' Vincent suggests.

'Naked time,' someone from Wendy's audience declares.

When she turns to see who has spoken, Wendy discovers most of the women from her audience are already undressing and she is one of the few left wearing clothes.

Vincent and Wendy have been involved in swinging for the last six years of their marriage. Annually they host three or four parties and attend roughly one each month at venues throughout, and just outside, the Nottingham area. Juggling their status as parents, making sure their children are in the company of appropriate grandparents, they swing with a small circle of friends who also host their own private parties.

Rather than making a joint decision to get into swinging, Vincent says, 'It just seemed to happen.' One night, at the end of a party with close friends, he explains that they simply found themselves having group sex. It didn't seem extraordinary and all the participants (three couples, including themselves) decided they should play together on a regular basis. The arrangement has continued in an organised fashion, and the clique regularly try to expand their circle of swinging friends by introducing interested couples to their group.

This evening, at Wendy's instruction, the four couples with whom they regularly swing have each been instructed to bring another couple.

The summery blonde loses her skirt and lies down on the lawn. Another woman, Wendy's close friend Mary, dips her head between the blonde's legs. The impromptu show of lesbian sex gathers a small audience as Mary licks and tongues at the blonde with passionate enthusiasm.

The fear of being seen is not a consideration, as the privacy of Wendy and Vincent's landscaped garden is guarded by a hedge of tall trees and a comfortable distance from the nearest neighbours. When another couple join Mary and the blonde on the lawn – this time it's a man and a woman, stroking, caressing and intimately exploring each other – no one is worried that their outdoor fun is going to cause offence or unwanted interest.

It doesn't take long before two men are helping another woman out of her clothes and guiding her to a convenient stretch of the lawn near the first two pairs of lovers.

Vincent kisses his wife again before heading over to watch Mary and the summery blonde. Wendy turns to the only other couple who have not attempted to join in the activities and begins to apologise for her jokes at their expense.

Speaking after the party, Vincent and Wendy confess that they can usually guess a swinger's occupation, marital status and financial income purely from a glance at their naked body. Considering the enthusiasm with which they discuss the subject, it is apparent that this game is a large part of the entertainment they enjoy at each party and almost as important to them as the freedom they achieve through their swinging.

'Mothers are easy to spot,' Wendy says, ticking examples off on her outstretched fingers. 'Stretch marks and paunches are hard to hide unless they've really been working out at the gym or, more usually, unless they're wearing a really broad suspender belt. Even then, it's usually only the mothers who wear the really broad suspender belts. I suppose that makes the item a little like having a tattoo that says "I am a mother."'

She draws a deep breath before hurrying on with her explanation. 'On the subject of tattoos, those girls who have blue-ink tattoos on their wrists are usually receiving benefits.'

Vincent calls his wife a snob.

Wendy sniffs, says wrist tattoos are indicative of adolescents who 'aspire to be Davina McCall when they leave their council estate', and then she continues on her theme. 'At swingers' parties, you don't see many of those nice Celtic designs that girls have on their backs, just above their bottoms. But I think that's because they're usually on the backs of girls who have über-possessive boyfriends. I suspect the design has been put there so he can follow the mazelike design while he's taking her doggy-fashion. To that sort, it's the mental equivalent of *The Times*' crossword.'

Despite a resolve not to encourage his wife's superciliousness, Vincent laughs.

'It's the same with tattoos with names on them,' Wendy continues. 'It's almost as though the girl has been branded. I can't recall seeing more than a dozen "name" tattoos in all the time we've been swinging.'

Clearly embarrassed by Wendy's superior attitude, Vincent interrupts his wife and tries to steer the conversation back towards less contentious areas. 'You can easily tell people who work in hospitals because they carry that hospital smell with them. There's an awful lot of nurses who do swing and quite a few doctors. I always get a smug rush of pleasure from surprising a naked girl while I'm kissing her and asking her which hospital she works in.'

'Yes,' Wendy snipes tartly. 'And then you ask them if they've brought their uniform.'

Unabashed, Vincent continues, 'Military types aren't as common, I've heard rumours that they usually sort out their own arrangements at army and air force bases, but they're the easiest ones to spot.' He shivers and adds, 'I can't imagine the training soldiers must have to suffer to constantly stand so rigid.'

'It promotes stamina,' Wendy interjects dryly.

Vincent ignores her. 'The training must be unbearable. They all stand as though they're out on a parade ground even when they're waiting in line for a gang-bang. Their backs are ramrod straight, stomachs in, chests out and shoulders squared and they look so stiff it makes you feel damned uncomfortable.'

'Stiff men only make me uncomfortable when they're doing it wrong,' Wendy quips.

Vincent does not reply.

At the party, Wendy is on a charm offensive. Darren and Julie (he works as an AO at the tax office, Julie is an EO and his immediate supervisor) have swung twice before. However, they have never previously been to a swingers' party and this is the first time they have allowed so many people to know about their penchant for swapping and recreational sex.

'I had no idea you two worked for the tax office,' Wendy lies easily. 'You must think my jokes were so rude and callous.' As she speaks, Wendy has one hand on Darren's arm while she smiles warmly at Julie.

The couple are at least fifteen years younger than her – twenty-five to her forty – but the age difference is meaningless in this environment. On the lawn, Mary is twenty years older than the summery blonde she is licking. Beverley, the woman sucking one erection while being ridden by another, is three years younger than the man in her pussy and twelve years older than the one in her mouth.

Wendy coos with surprise when she notices the breadth

of Darren's bicep. Enthusiastically, she congratulates Julie for having such a fine specimen of manliness as her husband. With an affected air of admiration, she asks Julie why the woman would want to share such a 'hunk'.

Not surprisingly, the pair warm to her. As the couple enthuse about their motives for swinging, their ambitions to build on the foundations of a good sex life, and their need to defy contemporary conventions in favour of leading the lives that they want, Wendy's comments about those who work in the tax office are either forgotten or dismissed as being unimportant.

'You two need to meet up with Kate and Ben,' Wendy tells them. After calling to a mixed-race couple – Kate is wan, with a very English complexion, while Ben's flesh is so black it looks like polished ebony in the dusk's fading light – Wendy explains that Kate and Ben hold identical views on the subject of swinging. She makes perfunctory introductions before leaving the foursome in an animated conversation. The temptation to stay with them is strong: Ben is handsome and there is something about Julie that stirs a warmth in Wendy's loins, but both couples are young and zealously defensive about their swinging. More experienced, and less inclined to waste a good party preaching the benefits of recreational sex to a converted choir, Wendy prefers to enjoy the physical pleasures of the party rather than listen to rhetoric.

Casually, she glides to the side of her husband and tells him she has made amends for her faux pas. Vincent is already involved in a threeway embrace between Janice, another new face at the party, and Derek, Beverley's husband. Vincent congratulates his wife on her diplomacy while Janice strokes his erection. Derek cups Janice's bare buttocks while pressing kisses into the nape of her neck. Vincent asks his wife if she would care to join them but Wendy politely declines and says she wants to 'keep an eye on the party'. Vincent smiles resignedly at her back as she disappears, certain that what she really wants to do is watch the newbies and see if her opinion on the taxman's cock will be proved correct.

Afterwards, Wendy says, 'Teachers seem to prefer organised games. Those sorts of shenanigans have never appealed to Vinnie and I. Organisation spoils the spontaneity and the tedium of sorting out games, and then expecting a group as unconventional as swingers to play by the rules, is more hassle than it's worth.' She sips at her latte, draws a deep breath and then, hurrying on with a caffeinated rush of dialogue, she adds, 'Povs tend to be defensive and pretend they've got money by wearing oversized CZs and plate jewellery. And those with money tend not to flaunt it, although you can always tell a genuine tan from those lurid-orange sunbed affairs. And it's easy to see who has the cash to afford cosmetic surgery because, when you're naked, it's difficult to conceal any scars.'

'Also,' Vincent breaks in, 'it's particularly easy to spot the snobs at our parties because she's usually the one hosting the damned thing.'

The couple glare at each other for a moment, and then laugh happily together.

The party looks like it will be remembered as a success. Dusk is falling over a lawn strewn with writhing bodies. Murmured sighs of orgasm and ejaculation can be heard beneath the second Norah Jones CD from Vincent's collection.

Wendy lies between the sweat-slick bodies of Don and Philip. The two men are close friends who have been swinging with Vincent and Wendy since the couple first found themselves involved in the lifestyle. Together, they have brought Wendy to a cataclysmic multiple orgasm when she had Don inside her pussy and Philip in her anus. Both holes are still slippery from the remnants of her own excitement and a liberal dousing of KY Jelly. Memories of the pleasure continue to tingle through her as she eases herself from between them.

Ever the thoughtful hostess, Wendy retrieves a glass ashtray from inside the house, as well as a silk robe that hugs her contours, and then walks carefully around the spent couples retrieving their used condoms and telling them that there are aperitifs available in the house. Some of the couples continue to play with each other as the last of the day's light fades from the sky above. The majority ease themselves from the lawn, collect clothes and discarded glasses, before stepping into Wendy and Vincent's home to have a final drink before going home. The only couples to remain outside are Kate and Ben and Darren and Julie.

When Wendy later tells her husband how she spent her evening with Philip and Don, she makes the announcement in the same matter-of-fact tone she would use to describe making a quiche with free-range eggs and organic peppers. Admittedly, her description excites him much more than a list of ingredients ever could but, for Wendy and for Vincent, her experience of double penetration has not been the major feature of the party. It has been a good evening – invigorating, fun and rewarding – but, for Vincent and Wendy, the sex is never the most important part of a party. The total enjoyment, the freedom to be themselves and the freedom to enjoy themselves in a way that best suits their needs are the most vital elements.

'I don't think there is any section of society that doesn't swing,' Wendy confides. 'Beverley and Don have been with their plumber and his wife several times. She's also done her regular mechanic, although he's single, so I'm not sure if that counts. But I know she said she was trying to persuade their regular builder and his wife to go away with them for a weekend. However, that's Beverley and she does like her rough and ready C1s and C2s. Her husband's a surgeon, so, I'm thinking, she has a thing for the different feel you get from callused hands.' She laughs, a high-pitched sound that cuts off quickly, before adding, 'I suppose I ought to try one myself before dismissing them. But our parties seldom seem to attract the working classes.'

Vincent says farewell to Janice and Peter, the second couple to leave. They have been entertaining, open and exciting and he is not offering false hope when he promises to send them an invitation to the next party. He returns to the remainder of the guests who are standing at the patio windows and casually watching Kate, Ben, Darren and Julie. The foursome have been writhing together for the best part of two hours and there are no signs of their tiring. From what started as a simple exchange of partners (Ben going with Julie and Darren going with Kate) they have moved on to Julie going with Kate, Kate going back to Ben, and now the four of them are joined together with the two women in a 69 position while Darren and Ben each take their own wives from behind.

'They're very energetic,' Beverley muses.

'If they stay there much longer, the grass beneath them will turn yellow,' Wendy replies.

The remark earns a chuckle from Vincent and Don.

Mary, Derek and Philip are away from the window and discussing a potential business arrangement. The seriousness of their conversation is the antithesis of the licentious revelry they were all enjoying earlier. Derek makes a reference to his legal team's agreement and Mary promises to email appropriate marketing projections. Philip seems to be the only one who remembers that they are attending a party. Without moving from his seat with the other two, he calls and asks why they are watching the foursome.

'Wendy's bet me a case of *nouveau* that the taxman will have a small willy,' Beverley explains. She speaks without snatching her gaze away from the window.

'How appropriate that you're betting for *nouveau*,' Derek remarks dryly. 'I wouldn't have thought this wager involved anything mature.'

Wendy chuckles, and she can see that Beverley wants to

grin at Derek's clever put-down. Instead of laughing with him, Beverley tells Derek to go back to talking business.

She turns back to glance out of the window and then squeals with obvious disappointment. 'Damn!' she exclaims, watching Kate and Ben and Darren and Julie extricate themselves from each other. Frowning at Wendy, she says irritably, 'It looks like I owe you a case of *nouveau.*'

'It's not that people are cagey about revealing their occupations when they're at swingers' parties,' Vincent explains. 'Aside from the sex, and the social side of swinging, I've known couples use parties to build themselves some strong business contacts. But, because everyone fears being named and shamed, it always seems as though a person's occupation is the last detail to be revealed.'

'I never know if that's a good thing,' Wendy complains. 'I don't know if those people are doing business because it's almost like some unspoken form of blackmail. I often wonder if they're doing business with fellow swingers because there's the constant worry that, if you don't do business with the people you swing with, they'll let your other customers know that you and your wife are a pair of perverted swingers.'

Vincent considers this and then shrugs. 'Wendy isn't naturally a cynic but she's working hard to become one.'

'I'm just saying,' Wendy complains. 'Swinging parties can be a lot of fun but there are some unscrupulous bastards who turn up as well as the decent people.' On the subject of unscrupulous people she explains, 'There are some people who are just out for what they can get. I suppose it should be expected in an atmosphere where people are meeting to have sex with each other, especially when it's supposed to be no strings attached and no questions asked. But we prefer our parties to be more relaxed and it can spoil the atmosphere if you're constantly on your guard for the creeps.'

Nodding, Vincent says, 'Some couples are just out for the fast fuck. If that's what you're into, then that's great. But Wendy and I try to build a little bit of a relationship with a couple before we get down to business. We've been lucky with the way we got into swinging but you hear so many horror stories of time-wasters, picture collectors, wankers and general scum that, I imagine, it could really sour one's disposition towards the lifestyle. Also, you have to watch out for the occasional weirdo who brings along an unexpected fetish that no one has bargained for and there are also –'

'To simplify what my husband is trying to say,' Wendy breaks in, 'swinging isn't for everyone.' She grins wickedly and adds, 'Most particularly, it should not be for taxmen because they all have small cocks.'

Shelly

'Which one of us do you want first?'

I'll see you in half an hour,' Shelly promised.

It was the sixth and final phone call and, as soon as she had hung up, an agonising fist of nervousness clutched her stomach. The pain was strong enough to make her collapse into a chair. Her hands shook as though she was in the throes of a fever. Her throat was parched and arid, and she wondered what mad impulse had made her want to organise a gang-bang.

Her morning had been spent in a splendour of perfumed pampering. She had showered, shaved and cosseted her body in preparation for the forthcoming afternoon. As she sat on the side of the bath, a shapeless dressing gown concealing her feminine curves and a mud mask hiding her face, Shelly had idly drawn a Bic against her calves and then removed the last stray hairs from her bikini line.

And she had allowed her mind to remain blank. Throughout all of the preparations, she hadn't let herself brood on the reasons why she was grooming herself to perfection. Instead of thinking about what would happen, and what would be expected of her, she had simply considered the forthcoming afternoon as an impending surprise. Something was going to happen – something new and different and like nothing she had ever experienced before – but Shelly wouldn't let herself think about the prospect with any depth. In a fugue of self-imposed ignorance, she had luxuriated in a morning of glib preparations and pleasant recollections.

But, with the final phone call made, Shelly could no longer hide from the truth of what she was going to do. She was less than thirty minutes from meeting seven strangers and they would all expect to fuck her.

Panic and excitement combined to make bile rise at the back of her throat. Her stomach twisted. Her bowels churned. Her heartbeat raced and she was suddenly swathed with a slick and greasy perspiration. Shelly had quit smoking five years earlier – a present to herself to mark her thirtieth birthday – but she now craved a cigarette so badly she would have happily fallen back into her old habits and gone through an entire pack.

Her hands continued to shake as she tried to dress. The nervous shivers made her clumsy enough to rake a thumbnail through one stocking. The two-minute chore she had anticipated these final arrangements to be took the best part of twenty. There was little time left to admire the combination of stockings and short skirt, the tight top that hugged her breasts, or the heavy and obvious makeup. After glancing at her watch, and realising she was in danger of being late, she snatched up her car keys and bolted out to the Red Lion where she had arranged the rendezvous.

At the age of 35, Shelly understood that some of her friends believed she had everything. Her nursing career was progressing smoothly into the ranks of senior management, and the rewards had allowed her to climb high on the property ladder. The eighteen-month-old BMW she drove was her perfect car, and the portfolio of investments she had made in the 90s was performing surprisingly well. The fact that she had no husband, partner or regular lover made her colleagues and friends even more envious because they believed she was free to live her life exactly how she wanted.

But Shelly did not believe she had everything. And the assignation she had organised was her determined attempt to grasp something she had desired for a very long time.

She parked, surprised the Red Lion's car park was so much busier than usual for a Sunday lunchtime. When it crossed her mind that several of the vehicles were there for her, Shelly's stomach lurched again and she struggled against the urge to be sick. A tall stranger approached her car – she remembered she had described the convertible BMW to all the participants and promised the hood would be down regardless of the weather – and then he was tentatively introducing himself as Sean. They shook hands. Shelly thought it was a ridiculously formal greeting considering what they were intending to do, and she gave Sean a small kiss on the cheek. She was tempted to press her lips against his, and possibly force a French kiss on him, then decided that would be too much for a welcome. Seeing another pair of strangers approach, she stepped back from Sean and forced a cheerful greeting as she waved for them to join her. One man walked out of the Red Lion's front door, adding to the exodus that bore down on her. Three more strangers climbed easily from their cars and made for Shelly's BMW.

Technically, Shelly told herself, the men weren't strangers. It was true that they had never physically met each other before but she had communicated with six of them through the internet prior to organising this event.

Introductions were made; so many of them that Shelly forgot the names almost as soon as they were made. Aside from Sean, she heard mention of Lee, Matt, Nigel, Oliver, Paul and Ray.

'Should we all have a drink to help you calm down?' Sean suggested.

Shelly could have hugged him for being so thoughtful and she nodded eagerly. Allowing the gang to herd her towards the pub, she ordered a double vodka in the hope it would help to soothe her anxiety. The men were cheerful and easy going, their gazes were appreciative and their smiles were filled with a knowing promise that finally ignited her arousal. The knowledge that she was so close to having sex with all of them was a powerful aphrodisiac. One man touched her thigh while she chatted with another. Another was deliciously tactile, stroking her hand and allowing the contact to linger far longer than necessary. Shelly downed a second double vodka, then said they should take the party back to her place.

As soon as she had spoken, she realised she had committed herself to the gang-bang.

All her initial anxieties returned with more force than ever. If it hadn't been for a personal promise not to go into this drunk, she would have tried to steady her nerves with a third double vodka.

The journey to her home was made in her BMW and two of the other cars. Shelly didn't particularly care whether her neighbours knew what she was doing but she didn't want to draw attention to her activities by having six cars parked along the avenue in the middle of a Sunday afternoon.

The seven men should have been eight but yesterday evening two of her initial guest list had said circumstances had worked against them and they wouldn't be able to attend. Because she wanted as many men as possible for this afternoon, Shelly had contacted all of the others and asked if any of them could bring a friend or two. With a little more notice, she believed she could have had as many as two dozen guys at her disposal. But, because her call went out so late, only Matt was able to solicit the help of his friend Oliver.

She brought tins of beer from the kitchen when they were back at her home – two cases of Carlsberg that she had purchased especially for this afternoon – and gave directions to the lavatory for when they would be needed. Turning the radio on to Jazz FM, and increasing the volume so it was just a little louder than she normally enjoyed, Shelly watched the strangers drink her beer and realised they were all hesitating and waiting for a signal to begin.

'OK,' she said, taking charge of the room. 'The rules are simple and I trust you'll all abide by them.'

The seven regarded her with respectful silence.

'Condoms will be worn at all times. If I say no, it means no. You can use my face and my pussy, but not my arse. Other than that, all I expect you to do is make me have a good time.'

She shrugged off the jacket she had been wearing to reveal her tight skimpy top. Her breasts were almost spilling from the scooped neckline and the fabric hugged close enough to display the rounded swell of each orb and the eager thrust of her nipples. Daringly, knowing they were all watching, she teased herself through the fabric. Her nipple stiffened obviously. Noticing the reaction her bold behaviour was arousing – the strangers had their attention fixed on her, some of them adjusting their pants, a couple of them licked their lips – Shelly pulled one breast free from its confines. She pinched the nipple between her fingertips and sighed loudly. The pleasure was strong. The satisfaction of knowing how much the seven men wanted her was even more intense. While blushes of embarrassment warmed her cheeks, she was more aware of the fluid thrill that seared through her crotch.

Sean coughed, cleared his throat and asked, 'Which of us do you want first?'

Shelly regarded him coolly, as she continued to play with her breast. 'I'll leave that for you boys to decide.' After a moment's reflection, she added, 'Although I'd always thought, in these circumstances, the first one to get inside was usually the fastest one to get his cock out of his pants and into the girl.'

The comment broke the hesitation that had held them all. Matt and Lee were out of their seats, forgetting their tins of beer as they each made straight for her. Oliver and Ray were close behind, quickly followed by Nigel, Paul and

Sean. Someone kissed her mouth; someone else helped her out of her top; others touched her legs and bare torso. So many hands now held her body – lifting her, teasing her and carrying her – that Shelly couldn't distinguish one man from another. The strangers had become a single-minded gang and they worked together to guide her to the settee and remove her skirt and panties.

The sensation of vulnerability was not something she had expected. Nevertheless, as the smell of seven beery men became all that she could breathe and Shelly realised the moment of the gang-bang was now upon her, she was shaken by the fear that the control was no longer in her hands. If the group of strangers collectively decided they wanted something that she didn't, Shelly doubted her previously recited rules would dissuade any of them.

Callused fingers parted her legs. Someone touched her pussy and a shiver of anticipation made her moan. Through the crowd of faces around her, she saw the men were undressing. Her gaze fell automatically to their groins and she smiled at the sight of the hard cocks she had inspired. As a nurse, she was familiar with the sight of penises and did not usually find the sight of them to be particularly inspiring but knowing that she had made all of these cocks hard caused a rush of glorious pride.

A mouth was wrapped around her left breast and suckled lightly against the stiff tip of her nipple. Two hands kneaded her right. The day was darkened by the shadows of the near-naked strangers standing round her. Her ankles were pulled wide apart and then someone was trying to thrust his cock into her pussy.

The idea of a gang-bang had always been one of Shelly's biggest turn-ons but, because the fantasy was so extreme, it wasn't something she had shared with many people. Her last serious boyfriend had condemned the idea as sick and twisted, so Shelly had never raised the subject with him a second time and baulked at the idea of asking him to help her arrange such an event.

Prior to him, she had been with a lover who used the fantasy as fodder for their foreplay. He had told her how much she would enjoy being used roughly by a dozen or so strangers and Shelly had always found the idea intoxicating. However, before she had ever found the courage to ask him to help her realise the fantasy, their relationship had ended. And, while it had remained at the back of her mind as an accompanying scenario to the most intense sessions of her masturbation, Shelly had never thought she would ever turn that wettest dream into a stark reality.

'And then I caught five minutes of one of those talk shows,' she explained. 'I can't remember if it was *Tricia*, *Sally Jessy Raphael* or *Ricki Lake*. It was just some crap that came on after I'd finished watching the morning news on TV. I'd just been in the shower, and I was fingering myself at the time, so the fantasy of a gang-bang was at the forefront of my mind. I heard someone give the advice that, 'any woman could do anything if she put her mind to it', and I realised I could have the gang-bang I wanted if I just organised it for myself.'

Her simple explanation brushes over the complex details of visiting a score of internet chatrooms, surreptitiously making her desires known to strangers and assessing their suitability for what she wanted.

Nevertheless, after two months of planning, the arrangements proved successful. On a Sunday afternoon, her nerves appeased by two double vodkas and her arousal heightened by the lust of seven strangers, Shelly was on the verge of basking in her gang-bang.

The first shaft slid into her and she groaned. All her clothes had been removed save for her stockings and heels. Too many hands held her, touching her breasts, pulling her head this way and that so she could be kissed by either Lee or Matt or Oliver or Ray. She was still unable to properly place the name to the face and, in a fit of giddy excitement, realised she didn't properly know the name of the man who was fucking her. The thought made her sex muscles convulse hungrily as he continued slamming himself between her legs.

He came with a vulgar curse and a cheer of approval from his colleagues.

A second man replaced him – the first slipped out of the room to dispose of his condom and get himself a fresh beer – and Shelly found herself being twisted on to all fours so she could be taken from behind.

A brief spike of panic turned her cold as she realised her backside was now exposed to the man. Anal sex had never been something she enjoyed, which was one of the reasons she had stipulated no rear-entry sex when laying down the rules. However, because she was now at the mercy of seven horny men, she realised that her rules would have little sway if any of them decided they wanted to take her that way.

And she didn't know if it was the idea of being used against her will, an untapped interest in anal intercourse or simply the excitement of the moment. Whatever the cause, Shelly groaned through her first orgasm of the day as the second man erupted inside her. She could feel his erection pulsing against her stretched muscles and was relieved to find the climax met with another cheer of approval. As the second man pulled himself out of her, to be replaced by a third, she found a sheathed erection was being pushed into her face.

Greedily, Shelly accepted the length into her mouth. The sex was frenzied, rough and brutal. After her first climax she was overwhelmed by a barrage of multiple orgasms. The taste of the sheathed cock in her mouth was at once nauseating and stimulating. She could feel the warm and pulsing flesh beneath the antiseptic flavour of the prophylactic. She sucked hungrily as she gave herself over to the moment and reached out to touch some of the naked flesh that crowded around her.

The third man erupted. Another spasm of pleasure shook through her, and then something huge was being forced against her sex. She glanced down and was horrified to see that Oliver had the largest erection she had ever encountered.

With all the other men, Shelly had been able to judiciously acquire clothed and unclothed photographs over the internet. Part of her selection process had been based on the fact that each man had an adequate-sized penis but nothing too large. Yet Oliver's erection was formidable.

Matt's friend, Oliver, had been called in at the eleventh hour. He wielded eleven inches of thick hard cock. Shelly's eyes widened in horror as she guessed the penis was probably as thick as her wrist and, even though her sex felt slippery from enjoying the climaxes of the first three men, she didn't believe she was sufficiently wet, loose or lubricated to accommodate such a massive erection. 'I don't think I can fit you in,' she gasped.

The group turned her over and, in that moment, Shelly realised she was under their control. Strangers held her arms down. Two men forced her legs further apart. A hand went across her mouth, staunching her protests and almost suffocating her as it stopped her ability to breathe. And Oliver's monstrous cock continued to press at her sex.

The labia were pinched against her pelvic bone. The enjoyment had been wrenched from the afternoon as sheer terror took its place. Shelly's mood of saucy sexual adventure was replaced by a dread of cold uncertainty. She struggled to break free, twisted and turned her head in a bid to escape the hand at her mouth, and Oliver continued to push into her.

Tears poured down her cheeks. In the panic of the moment, Shelly didn't know if they came from terror, upset or pain. She could feel the others pushing her on to Oliver's cock and pure fright took over. If there had ever been any thought that the gang was there for her pleasure, it was now long forgotten and dismissed as the most fatuous thought she had ever entertained. The hands at her arms and shoulders gripped tight and hurt. The force with which they all held her was overwhelming and inarguable. But the most frightening aspect was the monstrous erection that continued to push at her sex.

She knew it was too wide. Accepting Oliver's shaft would be something akin to being fisted and the thought heightened her panic. But his fantastic length was another consideration that she didn't want to think about. The fear of being stretched, torn and injured made her want to scream. But she knew there was little hope of being able to escape as the rest of the gang held her steady and forced her against him.

With a violent lunge, Oliver was inside her. She shrieked, amazed that her body could accept his thickness and surprised that she still had the capacity to feel pleasure. He pushed inside with brutal force. As soon as the thick, fistlike head had pushed past her labia, he slid into her with a vigorous speed. All eleven inches sank deep into her overstretched sex.

Shelly's absolute terror was forgotten as quickly as it had arrived. When the hand was moved from her mouth, and the others warily released their hold on her arms, Shelly growled with satisfaction and rode herself back and forth along Oliver's huge erection. Panting, breathless, and chilled by the sweat covering her body, Shelly allowed Oliver to take her to a sudden and painful climax. His thickness continued to pound between her legs as she crested wave after wave of glorious satisfaction. When he finally came inside her, the sensation of his vast shaft pulsing was enough to make her wail. In a frenzy of arousal, Shelly continued to ride herself along Oliver long after he had grown flaccid. When he finally pulled himself from her sore sex, the gang started taking her two at a time.

Each time an erection slipped into her pussy, another would push into her mouth. Shelly sucked and fucked, writhing against each cock between her legs and rolling her tongue around the sheathed shaft in her mouth.

The conversation around her was a blur of vile language and coarse instructions.

She had a nice cunt.
Someone should be gnawing on her titties.
It was a shame her arsehole was out of bounds.

This last remark was followed by an inquisitive finger testing the resistance of her anus. The forbidden contact made Shelly shriek in protest. She slapped the hand away and was relieved to hear a grumbled apology. It was even more comforting to hear someone else (Sean, she discovered later) reiterate her initial instructions in a reproving tone.

The smell of sweat, semen and beer mingled with the stench of her own musk. Perspiration dripped from her brow into her eyes, blinding her so she couldn't see who was in either end. Repeatedly, she found herself alternately gasping, holding her breath and then drowning in a rush of climactic pleasure.

She snatched a drink of beer from one of the men, dribbling some of the contents on to her bare body to try and cool her feverish temperature. Lee lapped the spilt lager from her breasts, which encouraged someone else to chase his tongue against her sex.

A moment later, Shelly could feel a tongue against her clitoris while two cocks pushed at her face. Hands pawed at her back, buttocks and thighs. Her breasts were constantly kneaded, nibbled and sucked. And then she was manoeuvred into a position so one man could lick her sex while another pushed his cock inside.

The orgasms began to come with greater frequency and a much stronger intensity.

Oliver waved his massive length in front of her face and asked Shelly if she thought she would be able to swallow him. She shook her head and grunted an explanation that was meant to tell him he was too big for her mouth. Her throat was parched, and her head reeled from an excess of pleasures, so the explanation didn't come out with any clarity. Nevertheless, Oliver seemed to understand and said he would find somewhere else to put his erection.

Seconds later, Shelly felt her sex being stretched again as Oliver pushed himself back between her legs. This time she didn't need holding down to take him and she dragged her sex eagerly back and forth along his thickness.

'I don't know how many times they each came,' she said afterwards. 'Maybe two, three or four times. It wasn't something I cared about. I do know the experience was everything I had hoped it would be, even though it did leave me a wreck when they'd finished.'

The gang-bang came to a halt about three hours after it had begun. The last of the beers had been drunk. Two of the strangers (Ray and Paul) had already left. And Sean, the consummate gentleman of the party, was busy making sure Shelly was OK, while the others found their clothes and thanked her for the afternoon. They all promised to stay in touch and gave glib reassurances that, if she wanted, they would do this again.

For the week following Shelly's gang-bang, she phoned in sick to work and spent her days at home, lying in bed, hardly daring to move. There were bruises on her arms and legs. Her muscles ached so severely from the exertion that she spent the first two days crawling on her hands and knees. She had thought her pussy might be uncomfortable after enduring such an excess but she had not expected her body to feel as though she had competed in an iron-man marathon. After the stretching she had received from Oliver, Shelly found the inner muscles of her vagina were no longer as tight as they had previously been. However, the most frustrating side-effect of all was that she was simply too sore to suffer anything but the lightest contact for a fortnight after the event.

'Each time I remembered what had happened, I wanted to play with myself,' she says, laughing. 'But the thought of touching the sore flesh of my pussy was enough to make me wince. Ironically, every time I remembered why it was sore, I got another urge to touch myself.'

With a bittersweet smile, she says, 'I also had a lot of difficulty accepting what I'd done. I felt cheap and slutty and low. I don't know why I felt that way. I suppose it's because women aren't supposed to organise gang-bangs for themselves and enjoy the experience. Perhaps it was that, after the thrill of being so high, my metabolism needed to bring me down to earth. Or maybe it was just because I was totally exhausted and that can cause depression. Whatever the reason, I did harbour a lot of self-loathing. Even now, three months after it happened, I can't recall the day without blushing and getting stung by a pang of guilt.'

She also admits that, each time she does recall the day, the memories inspire an irresistible arousal.

'But I didn't like being held down. That part really did frighten me. And it's made me wary of organising a gang-bang again. I can understand why they held me down – I guess they knew I would get a lot out of having Oliver's cock inside me and, ultimately, I did enjoy it – but that element of the day was too close to turning nasty for my taste. If they had decided to use my arse, or go at me without protection, I know they could have done it just as easily and I would have been unable to refuse.

'Not that I'm saying I would never do it again,' she adds guardedly. 'I've seen Sean a couple of times since and we both talk about repeating the experience. I'd feel comfortable if he was there to help keep things orderly but, still, I know he's only one person. And it's so hard to find a dozen respectable strangers who are willing to participate in a gang-bang.'

Arthur & Betty
'. . . being a cuckold excites me . . .'

Although he is officially retired from chartered surveying, Arthur continues to provide some consultancy services to his former employer. He has invested wisely over the years and owns a delightful house in the village to which he had always wanted to retire. One of the downstairs rooms has been converted into a small but very functional office and, although he is fast approaching his seventies, Arthur has taught himself to make use of the modern technology. The 21-inch screen of a TFT monitor dominates his desk. The plain-paper fax machine occasionally whirrs into life, noisily spewing out a printed sheet, and his email software sporadically announces the arrival of his mail.

His in-tray is stacked with formidable bundles of property-related paperwork. A handful of bulging FEDEX envelopes sits in his out-tray. On the leather-topped surface of his desk a sheaf of curled pages awaits his immediate attention. And, instead of looking at his work, Arthur can only concentrate on the sounds of ecstasy that come from the room above him.

'I'm coming. I'm coming. God. Yes! I'm coming.'

'Betty's very vocal when she's having sex,' Arthur explains. His smile suggests embarrassment but the light in his eyes is not exactly shame and it is certainly not apologetic. He speaks of his wife with the adoration of a newlywed, even though they will soon be celebrating their fifth wedding anniversary. 'She's always been very vocal. That's one of the things I love most about her.'

As though she has overheard Arthur's remark, and is doing it for his benefit, Betty screams again. It is a shrill and gratuitous sound and followed by the cry: *'Go on. Fuck me. Fuck me hard. Fuck me with your huge cock.'*

Arthur's leathery cheeks turn momentarily florid. Instinctively, he glances down to his lap and shifts in his seat. Finally raising his gaze, licking his arid lips and flexing a smile that reveals pearly white dentures, he straightens his back, takes a deep breath and says, 'I love it most when Betty tells me what she's been doing. That's the part I like the best. If you ask any voluntary cuckold, I'm sure they'd tell you the same thing. It's most satisfying when she tells me all the details.'

Betty is Arthur's second wife and fifteen years his junior. A photograph of her sits on his desk revealing that she is an attractive and well-maintained blonde. Her large breasts make her physique look bulky but it is clear she continues an effective fitness regime and the impression of excess weight is only an optical illusion caused by her more-than-ample bosom. The photograph contains nothing improper, but the glint of Betty's smile makes it easy to believe she is the same woman as the one upstairs demanding more satisfaction.

'Harder! Deeper. Yes. That's it!'

Arthur reaches into his desk drawer, removes a small pill from a packet in there and places it under his tongue. His cheeks have turned wan and his mood is suddenly serious and fixed on something other than our interview. After loosening his tie, he relaxes in his chair and indicates that we will continue momentarily. Light from the French windows of his office makes Arthur's complexion look parchment white and shows that he is perspiring, despite the room's mild temperature. Shadows from the lattice-work of lead diamonds on the glass fall dark across his pale face.

Betty's cries continue to reach into the room – *'Use me, you dirty bastard. I need to feel your cock all the way in there'* – and the tick of the clock marks every passing second.

'You could say my heart condition was the thing that allowed me to become a cuckold,' Arthur says eventually. The expression sits awkwardly on his face and it's clear that he is struggling to regain his self-control after a disconcerting episode. It is also clear that talking about his relationship with Betty is his idea of normality. 'The doctor warned me that erectile dysfunction was a fairly common side-effect, but I said, because I've got less than four inches to start with, I probably wouldn't notice the difference.'

His smile begins to look more sincere. His *bon mot* has the ring of a polished and oft-repeated witticism but there is never any suggestion it might be untrue. The attack, if it was an attack, is now behind him. He even manages a good-natured grin when Betty releases a guttural roar. Her cry is loud enough to resonate through the woodwork. The bedroom must be immediately above because the sound of squeaking springs is now a backing track to our conversation.

'Two months after I'd started on the pills, I couldn't get an erection.' He says the words calmly, without regret or upset. 'After another two months, we sat down to talk about what was happening. Or, more precisely, what *wasn't* happening. Betty thought it was the end of our sex life but we eventually worked it out that it could be just the beginning.'

He goes into further detail, coyly mentioning that Betty has always had a voracious sexual appetite and suggesting that he had never been fully able to meet her needs. He also explains how the options for treating his erectile dysfunction were severely limited. Viagra was advised against because of the nitrate-based medication treating his heart condition. The other alternatives included injections to the penis or unproven tablets that were still comparatively new to the market. Neither Arthur nor Betty believed the medical choices were tenable.

'When I told Betty she should take a lover, she scoffed at the idea,' Arthur remembers. 'She asked how I would feel if she was having sex with another man and I told her that the thought really excited me. She didn't believe me until I showed her that the conversation had given me my first erection in more than ten weeks.'

Like a lot of voluntary cuckolds, Arthur talks about his erectile dysfunction and other sexual inadequacies with such a commonplace manner it would be easy to imagine there is no longer a stigma attached to the conditions. He has always known his penis was small and ineffectual in both length and girth. His stamina has never been particularly noteworthy and his lack of longevity as a lover has always caused him acute embarrassment and frustration. Since he first started to court Betty, he suspected his abilities would be insufficient to satisfy someone with such a demanding libido. And the influence of the medication has proved him right.

'Betty was reluctant at first. My family and friends have all but called her a gold-digger. She thought, if she started to take a lover, that course of action would prove them right. I reminded her that she'd never cared about their opinions before and asked why she was letting it trouble her now. She finally agreed to try it, as an experiment. If it didn't work out, we agreed we'd just put the whole thing behind us and move on. If it did work out . . .'

He takes a breath and listens to another shrill cry from above.

'Didn't I tell you it was tight? Now go on and stretch it a little. God! Yes!'

'If it did work out,' Arthur resumes, looking pleasurably flustered as he continues, 'we said we'd take it from there.'

To transform Arthur's cuckold fantasies into reality, Betty contacted a former lover from the days before they were married. Ostensibly arranging to meet him for a drink, she came close to backing out several times before Arthur managed to push her into a taxi and thrust a twenty-pound note into the driver's hand.

'We were both shaken by the enormity of what we were doing. But I knew one of us had to act, otherwise we would both have backed out. Betty went off in her taxi, to her date, and I spent a horribly long evening alone in the house wondering what she was doing.' The expression on his face is hard to read. His tone of voice says this is a fond recollection but his features are as strained as they were before he took his medication. 'I didn't know what to do with myself for the whole four hours and thirty-seven minutes that Betty was out. I couldn't concentrate on the TV. I tried reading and couldn't make sense of the words on the page. When I tried to do some tidying, I broke one ornament and used air freshener instead of furniture polish.'

'You dirty bastard. You like that, don't you? Don't you ...' Betty's question tapers off into a roar.

Arthur raises his gaze to the ceiling with obvious appreciation.

'She came back and I immediately knew that she'd had sex. Her lipstick had been kissed away. Her clothes were hanging on her as though they'd been replaced in a hurry. And she brought with her a smell of someone else's semen that was stronger than her perfume. I took one glance at her as she walked through the door and all four inches stood instantly solid.'

His eyes are bright as he remembers the evening. He licks his lips before continuing and flexes another smile that reveals the even gleam of his dentures.

'But Betty refused to tell me what had happened straight away. She wanted a Scotch and a cigarette before she was ready to talk. She wanted to unwind for a little while and compose her thoughts. I was just about bursting to hear what had happened and she stretched out the torment until it was beyond unbearable. When I told her I was desperate to hear what she'd been up to, Betty pressed herself against me, touched me through the front of my pants, and said I wasn't in a position to demand anything. "I've just been fucked by a man whose cock is twice the length of yours, and he manages to get hard," she told me.'

He pauses to listen to his wife groan in ecstasy above. Shifting restlessly in his seat, he adds, 'She made me wait on her hand and foot for the rest of the evening, casually dropping hints about how big and hard he was; how many times he'd taken her to orgasm; all the different ways he had used her; all the different holes he had been in and how satisfying the experience had been.' Laughing quietly, shaking his head, he adds, 'I'd swear she got as much fun from teasing me as she'd had from being with Thomas.

'Eventually, when I was close to begging, she finally relented to tell me all the details. I had expected we would have sex, but Betty told me we weren't going to be doing that any more. Instead, she sat next to me on the settee and unfastened my trousers. She related what had happened while she masturbated me.'

It was a pattern of events that became a regular habit for the couple. Betty arranged to meet an old flame, making sure Arthur knew exactly where she was going and who she was going with, and then she would come home and stroke him to climax as she narrated every graphic detail. Occasionally, she would break her account to compare Arthur (unfavourably) against the prowess of the man she had been with. She assured Arthur that his penis was small and inadequate and his skills as a lover were negligible and bordering on non-existent. Quite often she would make Arthur touch himself while she took care of her own climax. Always, they would fall asleep locked in the passionate embrace that their new love life had provided.

'I can't explain why being a cuckold excites me,' he admits. 'It's humiliating and it should be an ordeal. My wife is sleeping with other men. She comes home from her affairs and tells me the most gory details. She ridicules me. She refuses my attentions on those occasions when I'm able to get an erection. But I wouldn't be lying if I said it's the most satisfying sex life I've ever known.'

The shriek from the bedroom above is almost like the final punctuation to Arthur's narrative. Betty's vocal exclamations from before had been strong and powerful but this final scream has the ring of a gratuitous and genuine orgasm.

Arthur regards the ceiling with an expression of satisfied bliss. The contentment in his features is tempered by a tranquillity that looks almost spiritual. It takes him a long moment to regain his composure and continue our conversation. But, finally, he remembers what we are discussing and apologises for becoming distracted.

Betty went through a small notebook of former boyfriends and likely acquaintances, seeing some of them repeatedly and always telling Arthur exactly what had occurred. Some of her friends introduced her to their friends and, by the end of Arthur's first year as a cuckold, he was proud to know his wife had a notebook filled with more than 75 names and telephone numbers of men who would happily satisfy her carnal needs. She now has a diary that contains three times that number and sees, on average, five different men each week. Their ages range between thirty and sixty. Some are single; most are married. All of them, Betty is adamant, have larger and more capable erections than Arthur. He blushes deeply as he makes this last admission but, even behind the haze of red that now colours his cheeks, his features are set with an obvious pride.

'She sees more married men than single men,' he confides. 'But I don't understand why. And I'm not in a position to judge them for being unfaithful to their wives because I don't fully understand the situation Betty and I have created. She's not technically being unfaithful to me, because I know every detail of what she's doing. But I don't think anyone who knows about our relationship would ever call her a faithful wife, even though she's doing this for our mutual pleasure.'

The situation clearly perplexes him and it is apparent that this is something on which he has often brooded. But it is also obvious that he has yet to reach any satisfactory conclusions. Brushing the matter aside, he adds, 'This is a special treat for me.' He nods towards the ceiling, where all the cries and exclamations have come from a moment earlier. 'Listening like this makes me feel as though I'm more a part of what's happening. Even better are those occasions when I'm allowed to watch.'

Few of Betty's lovers are open-minded enough to allow a man in his late sixties to remain in attendance as they become intimate with his wife. However, Arthur assures me there have been occasions when Betty has insisted he be allowed to remain in the room and watch.

'Every time Betty has told me about her lovers, I've created the image in my mind. I've painted a mental picture with the help of her words and it has always excited me. But those mental images aren't worth that –' he snaps his fingers '– against watching the real thing. The sight of another man's erection slipping into your wife's sex. The sound of her sighing as he excites her. The smell of her sex, and the stink of it after she's been used. The frustration and embarrassment of seeing her naked and in his embrace . . .' His voice trails off. He shivers. When he raises his head again, his eyes shine wetly and it is unclear if, or why, he has been crying. 'It's arousing,' he says firmly.

That final declaration is clearly as much as he wants to say about the experience.

Our interview is interrupted by a knock on Arthur's office door. Before he has a chance to reply, Betty bursts into the room jangling her car keys. 'I'm giving Joseph a lift back home,' she explains, pecking him on the cheek. 'And then I've got to do a bit of shopping. I'll be back in an hour or so.' Leaning down to give him another kiss, this one more intimate and leisurely, she adds, 'I'll tell you all about it when I get home.'

AFTERWORD

The last few months have been a blur of interviews, travelling and intelligent exchanges with some truly incredible people. Too many days have been lost in a haze of research as I've tried to absorb information, track down fresh sources and catch interviews with some very remarkable people.

But, while it's been hard work, it has been immensely satisfying.

As I mentioned in the introduction, the subject of swinging is one of our society's few remaining taboos. I won't sensationally describe swinging as 'the last great taboo' because, of course, there are plenty of other subjects that our intelligent and civilised society deems necessary to ignore in the hope they will simply go away and cease to exist.

But, after all my initial difficulties of trying to locate interview subjects, and then gather information for this book, I can vouch for the secrecy with which swingers veil themselves. And I can quietly marvel that any new members of the lifestyle are ever able to join its constantly swelling ranks.

With the exception of the boldest exhibitionists, most of us are guarded on the subject of our sexual tastes. Even amongst the swinging community, swingers are only comfortable discussing their lifestyle with other swingers. The fear of being branded different (or, more likely, twisted, kinky and perverted) haunts every individual and is supported by the social mores of keeping our private lives private.

The natural anonymity of swinging raises a lot of questions, which is why this book was laid out in a format of what, where, when, why, how and who. However, the queries thrown at me since I confided in friends that I was writing a book on swinging have made me wonder if I've been asking the right questions.

Q: *'If you're swinging, do you have to wear condoms?'*
A: *'You should. It makes sense. But not everyone does.'*
The majority of clubs insist that condoms are worn for sexual activity on premises but policing this goes beyond the practical. Hosts at parties will usually provide condoms, or state during confirmation that condoms should be brought. As with so many things in life, the responsibility falls on the shoulders (or other parts) of the individuals involved.

Q: *'Are all the women dead fit?'*
A: *'Some of them have small round bruises on their bodies where they've been pushed away by ten-foot barge poles. Others are so stunning they make your typical supermodel look like a toothless old bag-lady. The majority are somewhere between these two extremes.'*

Q: *'Do the women come every time?'*
A: *'Yes. It's a condition of entry to any club, party or private meeting that all the women have to have at least one orgasm prior to them being given permission to leave.'*

As you may have guessed, by this point, my enthusiasm for moronic questions had begun to seriously wither. But I was asked, on more than one occasion, if the women involved are forced into swinging by their husbands. According to some sources, it was the Americans who invented swinging. A camaraderie of US fighter pilots, during World War II, took the brave step of initiating random partner exchanges for private amusement. Whether this was done to take everyone's minds away from the high mortality rate that fighter pilots suffered is a detail that has never been recorded but, considering that one in three didn't make the return flight home, it does seem a likely cause. The selection process for their wife-swapping was governed by the pilots throwing keys into a cap, each wife taking one, and then spending a night with the owner of the key. This gave rise to America's nefarious key clubs that were popular during the 50s and 60s and set the trend for the stereotypical image of swinging parties.

Quite whether this means the Americans invented swinging, or are merely more candid about their involvement in the lifestyle than most other cultures, is a matter for debate. But it does suggest that, if the wives were happily selecting keys and sleeping with the other pilots, their involvement in swinging was not reluctant or coerced.

However, as swinging became more popular, its detractors continued to claim that wives were forced into the lifestyle by husbands who wanted to 'legitimatise their philandering'. There was even a saying amongst swingers, still popular up to the end of the last century, that proclaimed: 'A husband leads the couple into swinging but a wife keeps them there.' And, while this was meant to suggest the fulfilment of shared marital ambitions by those with different agendas, it also sounds like both parties are being led into something with an air of reluctance.

But those involved in swinging today say this statement is no longer true. According to those owners of swinging clubs interviewed in the process of making this book, membership is now most frequently organised and paid for by the female partner of joint applicants. Hosts of swinging parties confide that women are more likely to make contact and confirm booking arrangements. And, of the couples interviewed for this book, there wasn't one partnership that came across as anything less than 100 per cent committed to the concept of their swinging.

That isn't to say coercion does not take place. In any group of adults, you're bound to find people pressuring others for one thing or another. But it's insulting to the love and mutual respect of so many balanced swinging couples to suggest that the wives are only involved in the lifestyle because of domineering husbands.

In the section of this book titled 'Who swings?' I've outlined some points that show swinging permeates nearly every branch of modern society and has existed, on and off, throughout recorded history. But, as a variation on the question 'Who swings?' several friends have been asking, 'What sort of people swing?' The question is barked at me as though I can confide easy recognition of a type by virtue of the third eye they have in the middle of their forehead, or the T-shirts they wear declaring: WE SWING!

When I tell people that swingers are just regular folks, my questioners don't believe me. Being honest, I'm not sure I wholly accept that answer myself. When I say that swingers are extraordinary in so many ways, my questioners give me a quizzical look and want to know exactly what I mean by that statement.

Surveys indicate that the average swinging couple are aged between 35 and 55, usually white in this country, and have been married for ten years or more before they begin to discuss open relationships. But, as I'm aware, these details do nothing to explain what type of person swings. The truthful answer is a paradox. Swingers are nothing more than regular people – and they are possibly the most sexually exciting group anyone could ever encounter. Away from the parties, swapping and sex, they are simply aunts and uncles, mothers and fathers, neighbours, friends, workmates and drinking buddies. There is nothing about them that marks them as different from their non-swinging peers. They come in a variety of shapes, sizes and descriptions that range from skinny to fat (through svelte, athletic, muscular and chunky), and from downright ugly through to truly beautiful with all the million and one variations that lie between those two poles.

Yet, taken as individuals, speaking on their favourite topic, or relaxing at a party with other swingers, they show a knowledge of sex, stimulation and arousal that is superbly stimulating.

Perhaps the thing that makes them special is the fact that these people exude a sexual attraction that has been specifically cultivated to make them visible to other swingers. Perhaps it's because they are open and honest and, in most cases, non-judgemental. More likely, it's the delicious incongruity of Mr and Mrs Average calmly discussing her G-spot, his penchant for cuckoldry and their most recent foursome.

But, whatever the reason, the mysterious appeal of swingers is undeniable. Regardless of the fact that they keep the doors to their world closed, as long as adults are honest in their relationships, as long as couples are open about their needs and desires, the allure of swinging will continue to grow and draw more and more participants each and every year.